The Language of Caring Guide for Physicians:

Communication Essentials for Patient-Centered Care

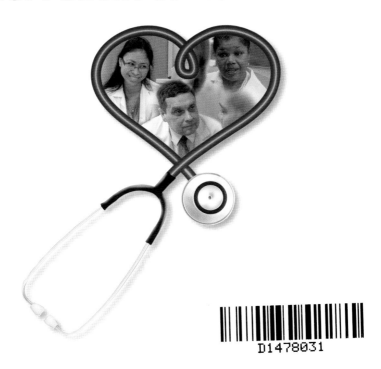

D1478031

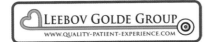

LEEBOV GOLDE GROUP
WWW.QUALITY-PATIENT-EXPERIENCE.COM

Printed in the United States of America

ISBN: 978-0-9882587-0–9 (paper)

Library of Congress Cataloguing-in-Publication Data

Leebov, Wendy and Rotering, Carla

The Language of Caring Guide for Physicians:
Communication Essentials for Patient-Centered Care

Includes bibliographical references

1. Physician executives

2. Physician Communication

Contents

Acknowledgments

We offer our heartfelt gratitude to the many people who contributed to this book's creation.

- To the patients, families, physicians and employees whose insights and experiences inspired this book.

- To the remarkable people at MD Anderson Cancer Center in Houston -- Ronald DePinho, MD and President, Thomas Burke, Executive VP and Physician-in-Chief, Ron Walters, MD, Asst. VP, Barbara Bowman, RN, JD and VP, Patient Services, Millie Hast, Program Manager, and Kay Swint, Clinical Administrative Director, as well as the talented physicians, staff and volunteers who served as the cast for the Language of Caring videos and the photos in this book.

- To the wise physicians who helped us discover evidence-based best practices and provided valuable feedback on early drafts -- Dan Arguello, Trina Bogart, Jeff Cohn, Kim Kahng, Tex Landis, Marcia Levetown, Jose Ma, Joe Miaskiewicz, Darren Shafer and Minisha Singal.

- To physicians Thomas Burke and Jeffrey Cohn who reviewed our book and wrote the much appreciated Foreword.

- To Ron Kalstein for layout and design, Nikki Gollub Bank for editing, Janet Kole for her wise counsel on intellectual property, Aline Rowens for literature search, and Sandi Guthrie and Scott Billingsley of Antenna Films for their masterful videography and photography.

- To the wonderful staff of the Leebov Golde Group: Nikki Gollub Bank, Chaim Bank, Linn Billingsley, Gabe Steerman, and Kelly Szymanski, for their far-reaching support and everyday encouragement.

- To Dorothy Sisneros and Jill Golde, our cherished Leebov Golde Group Partners, for their vision, for protecting our time, and for their communication expertise, feedback, care, and enthusiastic support.

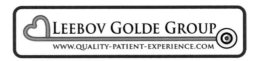

About The Leebov Golde Group

Driven by a passionate commitment to increase humanism in health care, the Leebov Golde Group helps healthcare organizations and healthcare professionals create and sustain healing experiences and positive outcomes through powerfully effective, caring communication. Leebov Golde Group clients include healthcare organizations large and small, including systems, integrated networks, academic medical centers, Veteran Administration hospitals, community hospitals, for-profit and not-for-profit hospitals, faith-based organizations, medical practices, longterm care and health plans. Leebov Golde Group clients have demonstrated breakthrough improvements in CAHPS performance and employee engagement.

About the Authors

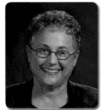

Wendy Leebov, EdD
wleebov@quality-patient-experience.com

A lifelong advocate and activist for creating healing environments for patients, families, and the entire healthcare team, Wendy Leebov has helped hospitals, health systems and medical practices achieve remarkable breakthroughs in the patient experience. Wendy is currently President and CEO of the Leebov Golde Group. Previously, she served as Vice President and change coach for the Albert Einstein Healthcare Network in Philadelphia.

A communication fanatic, Wendy has written more than ten books for health care, including three best-sellers. She also developed the widely acclaimed **Language of Caring Skill-Building System**, the powerful, video-based strategy that, by strengthening employee communication skills, dramatically improves the patient and family experience, as well as HCAHPS scores. Wendy also co-developed **The Language of Caring for Physicians: Communication Essentials for Patient-Centered Care**, the groundbreaking program that combines physician engagement events with video-based skill-building and peer coach development to achieve significant improvement in physician satisfaction as well as HCAHPS and CG-CAHPS performance.

Wendy's most recent books:
- **Physician Entrepreneurs: The Quality Patient Experience**; HCPro, 2008.
- **Wendy Leebov's Essentials for Great Personal Leadership**; AHA Press, 2008.
- **Wendy Leebov's Essentials for Great Patient Experiences**; AHA Press, 2008.

Wendy received her Bachelor of Arts in Sociology/Anthropology from Oberlin College and her master's and doctorate from the Harvard Graduate School of Education.

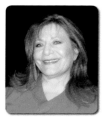

Carla Rotering, MD, MA
crotering@quality-patient-experience.com

Co-creator of **The Language of Caring for Physicians** web-based skill-building program, Carla J. Rotering, MD is committed to helping physicians create and sustain caring, healing, and gratifying relationships with patients and families, and with coworkers on the healthcare team.

Dr. Rotering is Director of Physician Services with the Leebov Golde Group. She practices Medicine and is Medical Director of Respiratory and Pulmonary Rehabilitation at both Banner Thunderbird Medical Center and the White Mountains Regional Medical Center in Arizona. With a distinguished background in leadership and education, Dr. Rotering was formerly Director of Critical Care, Chair of Medicine, and Chief of Staff at Banner Thunderbird. She currently serves as Chair of Professional Health and Wellness at Banner Thunderbird Medical Center and is a Physician Mentor for Medical Students at the University of Arizona College of Medicine, Phoenix Campus.

Dr. Rotering received her MD degree from the University of North Dakota School of Medicine. She completed an Internal Medicine residency at St. Joseph's Hospital and a Pulmonary Fellowship at Good Samaritan Medical Center, both in Phoenix. Dr. Rotering also earned a Master's degree from the University of Santa Monica in Spiritual Psychology, with an emphasis on Consciousness, Health and Healing. While continuing her clinical practice and medical leadership roles, Dr. Rotering conducts workshops, webinars and retreats for physicians, administrators, medical professionals and patients. She has co-facilitated Healing Path retreats for physicians with the Society for Healing in Medicine and the Grapevine Process for Physicians.

Dr. Rotering helps hospitals, systems and medical practices implement **The Language of Caring for Physicians** communication skill-building program with their medical staff teams. An expert facilitator and exceptional communicator, Dr. Rotering engages physicians with concrete skills they can use to enhance the patient experience as well as their own professional pride and satisfaction.

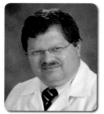

Thomas W. Burke, MD

Physicians care. We all came into medicine because we care.

But after more than 25 years as a practicing gynecologic oncologist, I know we can sometimes lose sight of that desire to provide for the whole patient.

Healthcare is a complex industry. In the rush of trying to get things done for our patients – having tests scheduled, reading charts, diagnosing ailments, and developing treatment plans – we may shift our focus to our tasks rather than to the person in front of us.

You want to respect your patients' time by moving quickly, but when was the last time you explained that to your patients? To them, you may seem distracted, hurried and even absent. When it comes to the patient's experience, perception is reality. Patients are vulnerable. Nothing heightens fear and anxiety for a patient more than the feeling that his or her physician isn't paying attention or explaining what you need to know.

In this book, Wendy Leebov and Carla Rotering remind us of the importance of communicating in a personal and empathetic way with the people who entrust us with their care. The straight-forward communication tools you'll find in this book remind us to connect with the people we serve. Everyone benefits. As a practitioner, I am more satisfied with my practice when I'm mindful and communicating with my patients and their families. And we know from patient satisfaction data that patients and their families value open, clear, and effective communication with physicians.

Listening to the voices of our patients results in improved outcomes and more satisfied patients. These authors make the salient point that we can't truly practice patient-centered care if we aren't practicing patient-centered communication. This means we can't effectively treat our patients unless we're actively listening, addressing concerns, inviting dialogue, and demonstrating how much we care.

In this book, you'll learn not only the skills to be a better communicator, but you'll find the evidence that supports the use of these tools. I hear from many physicians that they don't go in for touchy-feely programs that ask them to be something they aren't, and I would tend to agree with them. These tools, however, are grounded in testimonials from real physicians and, most importantly, in respected and peer-reviewed research.

I encourage you to be prepared to examine your current communication style as you read this book. I hope that, like me, before you reach the last page, you'll find yourself re-energized to engage with your patients and give them the best possible experience.

Thomas W. Burke, M.D.
Executive Vice President and Physician-in-Chief
The University of Texas MD Anderson Cancer Center

About this Book

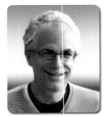

Jeff Cohn, MD, MHCM

The real owner of the healthcare experience is the patient going through it.

We as physicians have the opportunity to intersect with the patient along their journey and influence them in a way that meets their wants and needs. We are not captains of the ship. We sometimes have the privilege of joining patients on their journey and hopefully holding the steering wheel along with them to help them stay on course.

As we partner with patients, our communication skills are pivotal. Most physicians have been trained in a model that gives short shrift to communication skills. We apprentice. If we're fortunate to work with someone good at communicating, we learn. But many of us have only learned what NOT to do.

This Guide brings home the powerful impact that our language has on patients, families and colleagues. It identifies some of our glaring blindspots---words and actions that are well-intended but that have the power to deeply wound people. And it spells out in concrete detail the skills that are critical to partnering with patients and families and to shifting from physician-centered to patient-centered care.

About Dr. Cohn: Dr. Cohn is now President of the Plexus Institute--a community of diverse people – scientists, business executives, nurses, artists, teachers, journalists, researchers, physicians, college students, community leaders, and thinkers –united in their determination to foster the health of individuals, families, communities, organizations and our natural environment by helping people use concepts emerging from the new science of complexity.

Formerly, Dr. Cohn served as Chief Quality Officer at Albert Einstein Medical Center in Philadelphia where he was also a practicing Hematologist/Oncologist.

The Language of Caring Guide for Physicians:

Communication Essentials for Patient-Centered Care

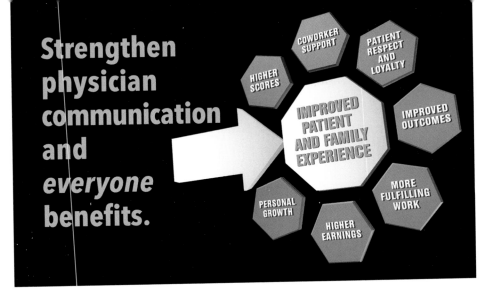

1. The Communication Solution

Physicians face tough challenges.

- Patients who are sick, in pain, anxious, vulnerable and feeling out of control
- Distressed families
- Patients and families with high expectations
- Consumer scrutiny -- with HCAHPS and CG-CAHPS scores on the web
- Hospital and physician pay-for-performance
- Competition for referrals and patient loyalty
- Extreme job stress and pressure
- Threats to professional pride and satisfaction
- …and change, change, change with Accountable Care Organizations, Patient-Centered Medical Home, organization-wide patient experience strategies, patient-centered care initiatives, productivity pressures, and more

These forces are making healthcare organizations and individual physicians increasingly accountable for positive clinical outcomes and the quality patient and family experience. And, all of these forces create stress and threaten physician quality of life and job satisfaction.

The Communication Solution

To thrive in this challenging environment, effective communication ---with patients and families, other physicians, students, and coworkers is, on your part, pivotal.

Public reporting of scores on HCAHPS and CG-CAHPS surveys make patient ratings of physician communication transparent to consumers, payers and peers. Consumers can post and find patient evaluations of physicians on line on more than 150 websites, including HealthGrades.com, Vitals.com and Angie's list. Also, most physicians are now on pay-for-performance plans that heavily weigh patient ratings of physician communication.

Patients are evaluating physicians on these communication factors:

HCAHPS

Doctor Communication

5. During this hospital stay, how often did doctors treat you with courtesy and respect?
   - ○ Never
   - ○ Sometimes
   - ○ Usually
   - ○ Always

6. During this hospital stay, how often did doctors listen carefully to you?
   - ○ Never
   - ○ Sometimes
   - ○ Usually
   - ○ Always

7. During this hospital stay, how often did doctors explain things in a way you could uderstand?
   - ○ Never
   - ○ Sometimes
   - ○ Usually
   - ○ Always

CG-CAHPS

How Well Providers (or Doctors) Communicate with Patients

The survey asked patients if their providers explained things clearly, listened carefully, showed respect, provided easy to understand instructions, knew their medical history, and spent enough time with the patient during the most recent visit.

Q16	Provider explained things in a way that was easy to understand.	
Q17	Provider listened carefully to patient	**Response Options**
Q19	Provider gave easy to understand information about health questions or concerns	• Yes, definitely • Yes, somewhat
Q20	Provider seemed to know the important information about patient's medical history	• No
Q21	Provider showed respect for what patient had to say	
Q22	Provider spent enough time with patient	

Also, the CAHPS Consortium has adopted several sets of supplemental items for the CAHPS Clinician & Group Surveys. Item sets are available to measure Shared Decision-Making and Cultural Competence of health care providers from the patient's perspective. These items focus on communication as well. For instance, take a look at the item set on Cultural Competence.

- Providers [Doctors] are polite and considerate
  - › Provider talked too fast
  - › Provider interrupted patient when patient was talking
  - › Provider used a condescending, sarcastic, or rude tone or manner with patient
- Providers [Doctors] are caring and inspire trust
  - › Patient could tell provider anything
  - › Patient could trust provider with medical care
  - › Provider always told patient truth about health
  - › Provider cared as much as patient about health
  - › Provider cared about patient as a person

While these items might remain optional, as the basic CG-CAHPS tools become required, practices with diverse patient populations are increasingly building them into their standard surveys.

Public scrutiny and pay-for-performance are not the only factors that make effective communication so important. Ineffective communication also leads to:

- Lack of patient adherence to care plans, post-discharge complications and readmissions
- Threats to patient safety, including medical errors and adverse events
- Lawsuits
- A less than stellar reputation
- Limited referrals
- Patient defection
- Sub-par pay-for-performance
- A patient-doctor relationship that is unsatisfying for physicians and makes the practice of medicine unfulfilling

The quality of your communication – the important spoken and unspoken conversations that reside between you, patients and families, and coworkers – has a far-reaching impact on outcomes, public perception, reputation, pay, job satisfaction and much more.

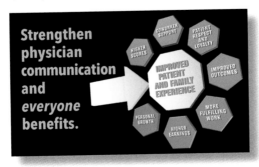

What Works? Patient-Centered Communication

The Institute of Medicine's landmark report **Crossing the Quality Chasm** (2001) identifies patient-centered care as an essential element of quality care.

IOM's 6 Aims for Improvement
SAFETY
EFFECTIVENESS
PATIENT-CENTEREDNESS
TIMELINESS
EFFICIENCY
EQUITY

Institute of Medicine. *Crossing the Quaity Chasm*. Washington, DC: National Academy Press: 2001

Patient-Centered Care: A Definition

"Health care that establishes a **partnership among practitioners, patients, and their families**...to ensure that decisions **respect patients' wants, needs and preferences** and that patients have the **education and support** they need to **make decisions and participate** in their own care."

Institute of Medicine. *Envisioning the National Health Care Quality Report*. Washington, DC: National Academy Press: 2001

In his plenary speech at the International Forum on Quality and Safety in Healthcare, Don Berwick, MD, defined patient-centeredness as "that property of care that welcomes me to assert my humanity and my individuality and my uniqueness and if we be healers, then I suggest to you that it is not a route to the point, it IS the point." In his **Health Affairs** article (***What 'Patient-Centered' Should Mean: Confessions of an Extremist***; July/August 2009), Dr. Berwick defines patient-centered care this way:

> "The experience (to the extent the informed, individual patient desires it) of transparency, individualization, recognition, respect, dignity, and choice in all matters, without exception, related to one's person, circumstances, and relationships in health care."

A pediatrician and professor at Harvard Medical School and the Harvard School of Public Health, Don Berwick, MD served as President and CEO of the Institute for Healthcare Improvement and Administrator of the Centers for Medicare and Medicaid Services. (Watch his compelling 3-minute speech on what patient-centered care really means at *http://www.youtube.com/watch?v=SSauhroFTpk*).

Please note: the Institute for Patient- and Family-Centered Care goes further to emphasize the vital role that families play in ensuring the health and well-being of family members. They acknowledge that emotional, social, and developmental support are integral components of health care. In this Guide, while we often refer to patient- and family-centered care, we primarily use the term "patient-centered care," because we believe that this powerful term includes attending to and authentically engaging family member's for the patient's sake.

The fact is, all definitions of patient-centered care require patient-centered communication with patients and their families in order to become a reality.

The Benefits of Patient and Family-Centered Communication

Patient and family-centered communication saves time and money, while improving health care quality.

- According to a meta-analysis by Indiana University School of Medicine, Regenstrief Institute, Centers for Disease Control and Emory University (Zolernik and DiMatteo, 2007)
  - › Effective patient-centered communication by physicians improves adherence to agreed-upon treatment and self-management of chronic disease, resulting in improved patient outcomes for diabetes, hypertension, and cancer.
  - › All but two out of 106 studies showed a positive correlation between physician communication and patient adherence.
  - › The patients of physicians who were good communicators were twice as likely to adhere to their treatment plans.
  - › Twenty-one physician training interventions on communication resulted in increased patient adherence. The odds of a patient adhering were 1.62 times greater if his or her physician had received communication skills training.
- Patient-centered communication results in fewer diagnostic tests, referrals and subsequent office visits. (Stewart et al., 2000)
- Patient-centered care is critical to addressing racial, ethnic, and socioeconomic disparities in health care and disparities in health outcomes (Society of Internal Medicine's Disparities Task Force; 2011 and Rao JK et al., 2007)
- Physicians who communicate well with their patients find their work less stressful and more fulfilling than those who do not. (Yi MS et al., 2007) Improved communi-cation has been shown to improve physician satisfaction and retention. (Pathman et al., 2001 and Suchman et al., 1998)

Selected References: Importance of Communication Skills

1. Bartlett G et al., Impact of patient communication problems on the risk of preventable adverse events in acute care settings. **CMAJ**;2008;178(12):1555–1562.
2. Beach MC et al., Is the quality of the patient-provider relationship associated with better adherence and health outcomes for patients with HIV? **J Gen Intern Med**;2006;June:21(6)661-5.
3. Bendapudi NM et al., Patients' perspectives on ideal physician behaviors. **Mayo Clin Proc**;2006;81:338–44.
4. Berwick DM, Improving patient care: My right knee. **Ann Intern Med**;2005; Jan 18;142(2):121-5.
5. Berwick DM, Definition of "patient-centered care." 3-minute YouTube video *http://www.youtube.com/watch?v=SSauhroFTpk*
6. Berwick, DM, Yale Medical School Graduation Address;New Haven CT: May 24, 2010;*http://www.linkedin.com/redirect?url=http%3A%2F%2Fwww%2Eapm%2Eorg%-2Flibrary%2Fpdfs%2FBerwickYaleMedSchoolGradAddress5_10%2Epdf&url-hash=hTG-&_t=tracking_anet.*
7. Essential Elements of Communication in Medical Encounters: The Kalamazoo Consensus Statement;**Acad. Med**;2001;76:390 – 393.
8. Levinson W et al. Developing physician communication skills for patient-centered care. **Health Affairs;**29:7 (2010):1310-1318.
9. Pacific Business Group on Health, **A CQC Guide to Improving the Patient Experience, California Quality Collaborative. 2011**;San Francisco, CA;*www.calquality.org*.
10. Rao JK et al., Communication interventions make a difference in conversations between physicians and patients: Systematic review of the evidence. **Med. Care**;2007;45(4);340-9.
11. Roter DL and Hall JA, **Doctors Talking with Patients/Patients Talking with Doctors: Improving Communication in Medical Visits**. Praeger: Westport, CT;2006.
12. Safran DG et al., Switching doctors: Predictors of voluntary disenrollment from a primary care physician's practice. **J Fam Practice**;2000;50(2):130-136.
13. Saha S et al., Patient-centered care, cultural competence and healthcare quality. **JAMA**;V.100, no.11;Nov, 2008.
14. Sutcliffe KM et al., Communication failures: An insidious contributor to medical mishaps. **Acad Med**;2004;79:186-194.
15. Yi MS et al., Self-rated health of primary care house officers and its relationship to psychological and spiritual well-being. **BMC Medical Education**;2007:7, 9.
16. Zolernik and DiMatteo, Physician communication and patient adherence to treatment. **Medical Care**; April, 2007;47(8);826-834).

2. Do You Employ Evidence-Based Communication Practices?

Through extensive literature reviews, the authors have identified seven competency areas key to effective patient-centered communication on the part of physicians. In your communication with patients, families and coworkers, to what extent do you regularly demonstrate evidence-based best practices? Complete and score the following checklist to establish your personal profile.

Best Practices in Physician Communication: Self-Scoring Profile

Best Practices in Physician Communication: My Profile *For each item, if you do this consistently, if your answer is "YES, I regularly do this," then put a check ✓ where you see the small box in the columns on the right.*	A	B	C	D	E	F	G
1. I acknowledge my patient's feelings in an empathetic way.				❑			
2. I take a deep breath and focus before approaching my patient.	❑						
3. I greet my patients warmly and establish positive rapport immediately.			❑				
4. When family members are present, I try to gain more insight about the patient from them.						❑	
5. When I have an issue with a colleague's actions, I address it directly with that person.		❑					
6. I validate or confirm the legitimacy of the patients' feelings.				❑			
7. If I have an issue with a coworker, I raise the issue in a caring way.							❑
8. Before I sit down with a patient, I prepare, so I can immediately show my knowledge of the patient.			❑				
9. When I'm visiting with a patient, I sit, lean in and adopt an open, receptive posture.	❑						
10. In hard conversations, I communicate empathy for the other person's feelings.							❑
11. I work together with the patient to set priorities for the time we have together.						❑	
12. I encourage patients to share their feelings.				❑			
13. When the patient is speaking to me, I pay undivided attention, instead of shuffling papers, typing, taking notes, or looking at the computer.	❑						
14. I ask the patient how much they want to know and honor their preference.					❑		
15. I open my mind to ideas and opinions from others on the care team even when they disagree with mine.		❑					
16. If a colleague has an issue with me, I listen and consider their point of view without being defensive.							❑
17. I avoid using acronyms and jargon, so patients can easily understand me.				❑			

Best Practices in Physician Communication: My Profile *For each item, if you do this consistently, if your answer is "YES, I regularly do this," then put a check ✓ where you see the small box in the columns on the right.*	A	B	C	D	E	F	G
18. I encourage the patient to speak freely about their concerns before I intervene.			❑				
19. I invite the patient's ideas and viewpoints before making suggestions.						❑	
20. I act as a positive role model for collaboration and teamwork.		❑					
21. I encourage questions as I proceed with an explanation.					❑		
22. I show empathy in my nonverbal behavior, by nodding and looking concerned.				❑			
23. I find out what people have understood, instead of taking for granted that they've understood me.					❑		
24. I make a concerted effort to engage the patient in decisions.						❑	
25. I check the patient's (and family member's) understanding and comfort with next steps before ending the visit.			❑				
26. When I have bad news to share with a patient, I plan my approach so I'm more likely to handle it well.							❑
27. When I'm with a patient, I am able to stop my mind from racing and really tune in to what the patient is saying.	❑						
28. I acknowledge and appreciate coworkers who are involved in the patient's care.		❑					
29. If family members are present, I show empathy for their feelings.				❑			
30. I make the last six seconds of my interaction with a patient a positive memory for them.			❑				
31. When family members are present, I invite their questions and address their concerns.						❑	
32. In a hard conversation with a colleague, I listen with an open mind to the other person's point of view.							❑
33. I find out from the patient what they already know, so I can build on this and address misinformation.					❑		
34. I communicate well with coworkers about the patient's care, so we will be on the same page and not confuse the patient.		❑					
35. When I'm with a patient, I make an effort to resist interruptions.	❑						
	A	B	C	D	E	F	G
TOTAL # of CHECKS IN EACH COLUMN							

How to Score Your Profile

Count: Count the number of checks you entered in the small boxes in each column and write the total below the column's letter in the TOTALS line at the bottom of the chart.

What do the columns mean? Your totals in each column represent the extent to which you regularly demonstrate best practices related to these key physician communication competencies:

Column	Competency Area	Your Score
A	Mindful Practice	
B	Collaboration and Teamwork	
C	Effective Openings and Closings	
D	Communicating with Empathy	
E	Effective Explanations	
F	Engaging Patients and Families as Partners	
G	Hard Conversations	

The checklist includes five items (best practices) associated with each of the seven competency areas and asks you to check off those that you employ regularly.

For each competency area, the lowest possible score is "0" meaning that you don't regularly employ any of the best practices for that competency area. The highest possible score is "5." A score of "5" indicates that you see yourself as employing all five best practices in that area of competency. The lower your score, the more opportunities you have for improvement.

Best Practices in Patient-Centered Communication: More about the Key Competencies

Grounded in extensive research on best communication practices for physicians, this book further defines and illustrates evidence-based practices related to each of the following seven competency areas.

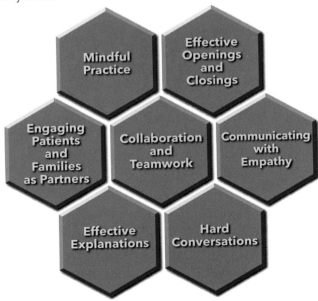

By strengthening and regularly demonstrating these competencies, you will exemplify patient-centered communication, which is key to providing the unparalleled patient and family experience and stellar patient outcomes.

About This Book

This book is a "how-to" guide to strengthening these competencies.

Competency	Highlights
Mindful Practice	• What is mindfulness? • The impact on the patient and physician experience • How to become more mindful: The discipline of mindfulness • Mindfulness and the Electronic Health Record

Collaboration and Teamwork	• Physician behaviors that interfere with team effectiveness and morale
	• Physician behaviors that inspire team effectiveness and support
	• Five strategies that foster effective collaborative relationships
	  › Acknowledge and appreciate everyone involved in the patient's care.
	  › Open your mind to diverse perspectives.
	  › Communicate with empathy in interactions with colleagues.
	  › Transfer trust during handoffs.
	  › Hold proactive conversations to ensure mutual understanding, harmony and cooperation.

Effective Openings and Closings	• The effective opening: Best practices
	  › Greeting the patient
	  › Showing knowledge of the patient
	  › Eliciting the patient's concerns
	  › Helping the patient tell their story
	  › Negotiating the visit agenda
	• The positive close: Best practices
	  › Checking understanding, comfort, and next steps
	  › Ensuring closure
	  › The last 6 seconds

Competency	Highlights

Engaging Patients and Families as Partners	• Physician behaviors that discourage partnership
	• Five physician strategies that engage patients and family members as partners
	  › Encourage the patient to speak up.
	  › Share responsibility for the direction of the discussion.
	  › Inquire and listen.
	    ¤ Help the patient tell the story.
	    ¤ Inquire about the patient's health-related beliefs.
	  › Use partnership language.
	• Engage family members too.

Communicating with Empathy	• The impact of empathic communication on the patient-physician relationship, the patient experience and clinical outcomes
	• The Heart-Head-Heart Communication Model
	• Specific techniques for communicating empathy
	  › The "Heart-Head-Heart Sandwich"
	  › How to acknowledge and validate feelings
	  › How to show caring nonverbally

Effective Explanations	*How to employ the state-of-the-art "Ask-Tell-Ask" model to provide effective explanations and ensure patient understanding.*
	• **Ask**
	  › Invite questions and listen.
	  › Elicit the patient's knowledge and concerns.
	• **Tell**
	  › Explain your positive intent—your patient-centered rationale.
	  › Use simple, easy-to-understand terminology.
	  › Watch patient's body language for signs of inattention or confusion.
	  › Invite questions along the way.
	  › Address anxieties and clarify "what ifs."
	• **Ask**
	  › Ask open-ended questions.
	  › Respectfully check for understanding using Teach-Back

Hard Conversations	• How to initiate and conduct an effective hard conversation, using the Hard Conversations Model • How to use the "Caring Broken Record" to hold your ground caringly when it's the right thing to do and the other person resists • How to respond to patient and family complaints with tact and caring

For each competency, you'll find:	Description
Quick Self-Check	• Begins with a short set of questions to help you zoom in on the extent to which you already demonstrate regularly those best practices related to the competency at hand.
Rules of Thumb	• Concrete guidelines gleaned from the evidence base identifying best practices related to the competency at hand • Illustrative examples for each Rule of Thumb
Highlights for Review	• A succinct summary of the Rules of Thumb and tips for effective skill use
Selected References	• A short list of books, studies and reports that provide an evidence base for the competency at hand • Expanded reference list at the end of the book
Self-Improvement Tools	• A Personal Spot-Check • Feedback tools for use with patients, family members and coworkers to tap their observations and suggestions regarding your skills
Reference Cards	• Cue cards with the Rules of Thumb on one side and, on the other side, a Spot-Check tool for reflecting on your effectiveness after a specific encounter
IN THE APPENDIX:	
Comprehensive Feedback Tools	• Unlike the tools in each chapter that focus on each competency, the Feedback Tools in the Appendix address all of the competencies together. • You'll find one for yourself, one for patients, one for family members and one for colleagues.
Comprehensive Reference List	• Each chapter includes selected references for that chapter. The Comprehensive Reference List at the end is much more extensive.

More about the Self-Improvement Tools

While simply reading this book can alert you to opportunities to improve, you will gain much more traction for improvement by consciously and conscientiously **applying** the skills after you review the Rules of Thumb described in each book chapter.

Suggestions

Try three-day experiments with one competency at a time.

If you concentrate your attention on repeatedly implementing the Rules of Thumb for each competency *for three days*, you will gain comfort with new behaviors. You'll experience the benefits and you'll begin building a *habit* of engaging in the behavior.

- Carry the Reference Card around with you for three days.
- Before each patient/family encounter, review the Reference Card and focus consciously on applying the Rules of Thumb in each upcoming interaction. After the interaction, answer the Spot Check questions on the Reference Card. This will take less than a minute.

Solicit concrete feedback about your performance from others.

It's not easy to be fully self-aware without feedback from others. While self-awareness and self-monitoring are critical, knowing how others perceive your performance can help you learn more about your behavior and its impact. At the end of each chapter, you'll find tools for inviting feedback from others, including patients and their family members, and your coworkers.

> Note: You may make copies of the tools you want to use, or you may purchase an **APP** for your phone, iPad or tablet that includes the Reference Cards and Tools. (For information, contact: *http://www.quality-patient-experience.com/contact-us.html*)

- **Obtain patient and family feedback.** Early in an encounter, explain the skills or behaviors you are working on improving. Alert the patient and their family members that, at the end of the visit, you will invite them to give you feedback about how you performed. At the end of the encounter, invite your patient and their family member to complete a short report card on your behavior. Ask them to drop their completed card in the box on the front desk when they've finished. Thank them for helping you become a better doctor.
- **Obtain coworker feedback.** Invite a trusted colleague to observe you and give you feedback. Provide them with the feedback tool at the end of each chapter.

Most people have blindspots about their own behavior and its impact. Feedback from others is invaluable in helping you overcome blindspots that might be interfering with your effectiveness.

All physicians can benefit from this book.

- If you're new to practicing medicine, this Guide will help you practice and master state-of-the-art communication skills from the start.
- If you're experienced, you can become even more effective and deliberate in effective communication and achieve even better outcomes as a result.
- And if you're already expert on communication, this Guide can help you become an even more effective role model, coach and mentor for colleagues and students, by fine-tuning and making explicit the skills and tips that derive from the latest research on the patient-physician relationship and patient-centered care.

The Man with the Saw

 There was once a man who needed to cut down a huge tree at the side of his house. He took his saw and he began sawing, as his teenage daughter watched. He sawed and he sawed and he sawed, and it seemed as if he was making no headway at all.

After exhausting himself sawing, his daughter said, "Dad, why don't you SHARPEN the saw, since it doesn't seem to be cutting through the tree?"

Her father replied, "I don't have time."

You may be swamped with work and pressure and feel that there's never enough time. By devoting short bits of your precious time to sharpening your saw---your skills and tools---, you will make your job easier, even less time-consuming. Consider focusing on one competency area every two to four weeks. Also, devote two minutes a day to reviewing one Reference Card prior to seeing patients for the day. By repeated review of the Rules of Thumb, you will become more alert to these best practices and first consciously, and then unconsciously, apply these skills as habit.

You will see better results with patients and feel more gratified in your caring work.

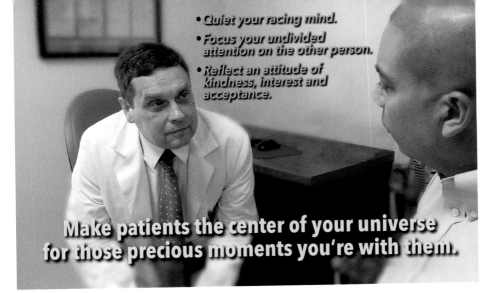

- *Quiet your racing mind.*
- *Focus your undivided attention on the other person.*
- *Reflect an attitude of kindness, interest and acceptance.*

Make patients the center of your universe for those precious moments you're with them.

3. Mindful Practice

🔍 QUICK SELF-CHECK	YES ✓
1. Do I take a deep breath and focus before approaching my patient?	
2. When I'm visiting with a patient, do I sit, lean in and adopt an open, receptive posture?	
3. While the patient is speaking, do I maintain eye contact?	
4. While the patient is speaking, do I remain quiet, listening and not interrupting?	
5. When the patient is speaking to me, do I pay undivided attention, instead of shuffling papers, texting, typing, taking notes, or looking at a computer or other tech device?	
6. If I'm interrupted during a patient encounter, do I resist the interruption or at least apologize to the patient before diverting my attention?	
7. When I'm on the phone with a patient or family member, do I focus fully on the person?	
8. When a colleague and I are talking, do I focus my attention fully on the other person?	
9. Do my patients feel listened to and heard by me when they're talking?	

A physician competent and effective at displaying mindful practice replies "yes" to these nine questions. "No" responses indicate opportunities to improve the patient, family and coworker experience by mastering and consistently using the skill of mindfulness.

The Mindfulness Remedy

Patients and families yearn for your full attention. If you don't tune in fully, they feel disregarded and perceive the interaction as impersonal. And they don't trust that you've heard their concerns and will provide quality care. Coworkers also value your undivided attention in interactions with you. They experience this as respectful and can more quickly handle the business at hand.

Of course, giving patients, families and coworkers your undivided attention is easier said than done. Facing unprecedented demands, most physicians feel the pressure of long hours, crammed schedules, new technology, documentation requirements and much more. Many long for greater fulfillment and relief from the stresses in practicing medicine today.

Your mindfulness is crucial for patients, families and coworkers. It also can greatly enhance *your* personal effectiveness and job satisfaction.

Mindfulness Defined

Mindfulness expert Jon Kabat-Zinn defines mindfulness as:

- Paying attention–undivided attention
- Staying on purpose (goal)--consciously
- In the present moment
- Without judging

Says Kabat-Zinn, only when you are mindful with patients will you release your innate compassion. He calls mindfulness "presence of the heart."

Mindful Practice in Action

Dr. Jeff Cohn's blog entry provides an excellent example of how mindfulness led to a surprising and potentially important piece of information that led to patient-centered actions owned by the patient.

Catching Butterflies (in memory of Jerry Sternin, PhD)

It was nearing the end of a block where I was serving as the attending physician on the "teaching service." One of my responsibilities was to evaluate certain physician-in-training skills through observing their interactions with patients. One of the first year residents asked me to watch him provide instructions to a patient being discharged to home. Mr. Johnson had entered the hospital over a week prior, having been admitted in respiratory failure due to emphysema. He had spent several days in the Intensive Care Unit on a ventilator, though he was now nearly back to his baseline status. The resident was convinced that this flare-up was due to Mr. Johnson not correctly taking his medication, and this was going to be the focus of his instructions. For over ten minutes, the resident spoke to Mr. Johnson in earnest tones about the importance of taking his medications regularly. He reviewed with Mr. Johnson how to take them reliably, reminding him what could happen (again) if this didn't occur. Mr. Johnson nodded in agreement; he had clearly been shaken by this hospitalization and didn't want a recurrence like this in the future.

At one point the resident asked Mr. Johnson to describe how he took his medications. Mr. Johnson replied, "Well, in the morning I usually take them before breakfast. Then I take them with lunch and dinner later in the day." The resident eventually reached the end of the interaction, provided the written instructions to Mr. Johnson matching those he had spoken about, and he then turned to me. "Do you have any questions for Mr. Johnson, Dr. Cohn?" "Well," I said, "I do have just one. Mr. Johnson, I believe I heard you say that you usually take your morning medications before breakfast. When I hear someone say *usually*, to me that means that sometimes it doesn't happen that way.
Is that correct? What gets in the way of you taking your medications before breakfast?" Mr. Johnson nodded and gave a sheepish grin. "You know, in addition to having emphysema I also have diabetes. So first thing when I get up, I take my insulin. And I know I have to have breakfast within 15 minutes or so or else my sugar will drop and I'll get sick. Sometimes one of my friends will call me on the phone after I take my insulin but before I take my lung medicines. I'll talk to him for a while and then I'll remember I need to eat some breakfast. So I'll get off the phone with him and make breakfast, and, I guess, some of those times I don't remember to take my morning lung medicines." "So, what ideas do you have as to how to prevent that from happening?" I asked. "I guess I should tell my friends that I can't talk if they call first thing in the morning and that I'll call them back after I've taken my medicines and finished my breakfast. That should do it, I think."

When Jerry Sternin of the Positive Deviance Initiative was coaching us years ago about how to facilitate "discovery and action dialogues" to come up with ideas and actions to prevent MRSA infections, he referred to the technique of "catching butterflies." One needs to listen with your whole self, particularly listening for the ideas that can be converted into concrete actions. As the ideas are spoken, imagine them to be butterflies floating up. The listener/facilitator gently catches them and holds them up to the individual/group, asking questions like, "What do you think? What could you do next?"

Jeffrey Cohen, MD

August, 2012
www.plexusinstitute.org

The Benefits of Mindfulness

When you're mindful with patients:

- You notice cues coming from the patient and gain invaluable information that helps you provide appropriate care.
- You ease patient anxiety, because patients FEEL your caring.
- You encourage patients to open up, to trust, and to partner with you in their care.

When you really listen, taking in whatever is arising, instead of trying to fix it, push it away, rush out of the room, or ruminate about the next pressing thing you have to do, this is profoundly healing for the patient.

And mindfulness is not all about the patient. Drs. Epstein and Krasner at the University of Rochester Medical Center have confirmed that mindfulness training for physicians has a powerful positive impact on care decisions, patient perceptions of their doctor and physician job satisfaction. You benefit from a stronger feeling of connection with your patients, greater patient satisfaction and loyalty, reduced stress, and pride in your positive impact on the patient experience.

Also, take a look at these HCAHPS and CG-CAHPS questions.
- How often does the physician listen carefully to you?
- How often does the physician spend enough time with you?
- How often does the physician treat you with courtesy and respect?
- How do you rate your overall experience?

When physicians become more mindful, patient ratings improve on these survey questions. Mindfulness helps you score high and this positively affects your reputation and your wallet --- under Value-Based Purchasing and pay-for-performance.

Mindfulness is learnable.

The good news is that strengthening your mindfulness skills is not hard to do. It requires the same kind of disciplined approach you've mastered in other aspects of your work and personal life, whether you become fully present when you do an invasive procedure or engage in an important personal conversation.

Rebbe Nachman of Breslav taught, a person can direct his thoughts wherever he wishes. And if they do sometimes wander, you can simply grab them and pull them back to where they should be. Just as when a horse strays from the path, you grab it by its halter and pull it back to the straight path, you can do exactly the same with your thoughts."

Based on Likutei Moharan 11:50; *Healing Leaves*, p.44

Distracted Doctoring: Avoid these behaviors that indicate an absence of mindfulness.
- Silence or non-responsiveness as you enter
- Lack of eye contact
- Turning to the computer or other tech device while the patient is talking
- Standing throughout the encounter
- Your hand on the doorknob
- Looking at your watch or pager
- Interrupting
- Texting while the other person is talking

Based on the Evidence: The Skills of Mindful Practice

 Seven Rules of Thumb: Mindful Practice Step-by-Step

1. Quiet your racing mind.

2. Take a deep breath. Bring your full attention to the present moment and the person at hand.

3. Sit. Lean in. Adopt an open, receptive posture.

4. While the person is speaking: Maintain eye contact. Be quiet. Don't interrupt. Don't think about what you're going to say or do next.

5. Avoid multitasking (shuffling papers, texting, typing, taking notes, looking at the computer).

6. Resist interruptions. Or if an interruption is necessary, stay present to the patient until you explain the interruption and politely disconnect.

7. Tune in fully.

"Yes, but...."

You might be thinking:

1. "Yes but how can I stay mindful when using a computer, notebook, phone or other tech device with a patient?"
2. "Yes, but I don't have time to spend more time listening to my patients!"
3. "Yes, but people interrupt me all day long. How can I give anyone my undivided attention?"

Overcoming the Obstacles to Mindful Practice

1. "Yes, but how can I stay mindful when using a computer, notebook, phone or other tech device with a patient?"

This IS a challenge! The fact is, many patients think the computer or other tech device damages their relationship with their physician. Some physicians stop making eye contact. Others, in their eagerness to get their documentation done in real time, disconnect from the patient before the patient leaves. The fact is, many patients feel anxious and even a bit paranoid when their doctor is using the computer without explaining what they're doing. And to patients, the interaction feels impersonal, even a bit dismissive.

You cannot effectively

Multi-tasking is

focus on the computer

very inefficient

and the patient

and makes patients

at the same time.

feel unimportant.

What works better? Studies at Kaiser Permanente have identified mindfulness as the best practice that ensures that tech devices will enhance, not damage your relationships with your patients. They advise against trying to pay attention to both the patient and the device at the same time. Multi-tasking is inefficient and patients experience you as disconnected and inattentive.

👍 RULES OF THUMB: Using Technology When You're with a Patient	
1. Log in and explain what you're doing.	• "Let's open up your chart so we have your history and results in front of us."
2. *Alternate* the focus of your attention, instead of trying to multi-task.	• Be mindful to the patient and then mindful to the device and back and forth. • Attend fully to one and then the other, instead of trying to attend to both at once. • When you ask a question, make eye contact. Don't be out of eye contact for more than 10 seconds. • When the patient is discussing an emotional or critical issue, turn away from the device completely and tune in to the patient. • When you're entering information, explain, "Please give me a moment to jot some of this down while it's fresh in our minds."
3. Engage the patient with the device and the information on it.	• Turn the screen toward the patient, showing there's no secret. Invite the patient to look on with you: "Would you like to look on with me? I'm reviewing your lab results." • Share information, like lab results. "Let's take a look at what the specialist note recommended from your visit last month."
4. Log in and out in front of the patient.	• Ease their concerns about confidentiality.

2. "Yes, but I don't have TIME to spend more time listening to my patients!"

No doubt, you have incredible demands on your time. The good news is that mindfulness does not take more time! In fact, it saves time. When you focus fully on your patients, you absorb what they're saying the first time they say it. You do a better job of hearing their concerns. You think clearly and provide more thorough and helpful care. And this leads to reduced phone calls, fewer return visits and better outcomes.

3. "Yes, but people interrupt me all day long. How can I give anyone my undivided attention?"

Interruptions are inevitable. And yes, they break your concentration on the patient and frequently cause patients to feel discounted. To prevent them and to handle them well when you can't prevent them, you will need to assert yourself.

👍 RULES OF THUMB: When Handling Interruptions

1. Tell your colleagues that you're committed to giving your patients undivided attention. Make it known.	"I want to focus fully on my patients when I'm with them. I'm working on staying mindful when I'm with them instead of trying to multi-task. I'm asking for your help."
2. Ask them to think twice before interrupting.	"For the patient's sake, I'm asking you to think twice before interrupting me. Unless it's an emergency, please wait until I've ended the patient encounter."
3. If you must attend to an interruption, don't slight the patient by turning away. Stay present as you politely disconnect.	"I'm sorry about this interruption. I need to attend to it and I'll be right back. I appreciate your understanding."

Wrap-Up

Patients want you to pay close attention---to listen ---to stay on point---in the present moment-- without judging. When you're mindful with your patients, you make the most of your precious time and you reveal your inherent compassion.

Highlights for Review: Mindful Practice

Pay undivided attention, on purpose, in the present moment--without judging.
  Jon Kabat-Zinn

👍 Rules of Thumb

1. Quiet your racing mind.

2. Take a deep breath. Bring your full attention to the present moment and the person at hand.

3. Sit. Lean in. Adopt an open, receptive posture.

4. While the person is speaking: Maintain eye contact. Be quiet. Don't interrupt. Don't think about what you're going to say or do next.

5. Avoid multitasking (shuffling papers, texting, typing, taking notes, looking at the computer).

6. Resist interruptions by others.

7. Tune in fully.

Don't let technology interfere with your relationship with your patients.
When using a computer, iPad, phone or other tech device:

1. *Alternate your focus!* Focus fully on the patient and then fully on the device in a back and forth fashion. Don't try to pay attention to both the patient and the device at once.

2. *Engage the patient.*
   • Explain what you're doing.
   • Share information.
   • Invite the patient to look on with you.

Selected References

On Mindful Practice

1. Greeson JM, Mindfulness research update 2008. **Complementary Health Practice Review**; 2009;14(1):10-18.
2. Gold J, Hospitals warn smartphones could distract doctors, March 26, 2012; http://m.npr.org/news/front/149376254?singlePage=true. Accessed October 24, 2012.
3. Krasner MS et al; Association of an educational program in mindful communication with burnout, empathy, and attitudes among primary care physicians. **JAMA**;2009;302(12):1284-1293.
4. Ludwig DS et al, Mindfulness in medicine. **JAMA**;2008;300 (11):1350-1352.
5. Shanafelt T, Enhancing meaning in work: A prescription for preventing physician burnout and promoting patient-centered care. **JAMA**;2009 Sep 23;302(12):1338-40.
6. Wang P, Gao F, Mindful communication to address burnout, empathy, and attitudes. **JAMA**;2010;303(4):330-331.

Mindful Practice and Use of Technology with Patients

1. Frankel RA et al., Effects of exam-room computing on clinician-patient communication: a longitudinal qualitative study. **Patient Educ Couns.**;2012 Feb;86(2):166-71.
2. Margalit RS et al., Electronic medical record use and physician-patient communication: an observational study of Israeli primary care encounters. **Patient Educ Couns.**;2006 Apr;61(1):134-41.
3. Nagy V and Kanter M, Implementing the electronic medical record in the exam room: The effect on Physician-patient communication and patient satisfaction. **Perm J.**;2007 Spring;11(2):21–24.

Self-Improvement Tools: On Mindful Practice

- **Personal Spot Check on Mindful Practice**
- **Personal Spot-Check on Using Technology with Patients**
- **Patient Feedback**
- **Family Feedback**
- **Peer/Coworker Feedback**

Personal Spot-Check: On Mindful Practice

With this patient, how well did I practice mindfulness?	YES ✓
1. Did I bring my full attention to the present moment and the person in front of me?	
2. Did I sit, lean in and adopt an open, receptive posture?	
3. When the patient was talking, did I maintain eye contact and listen, without interrupting?	
4. Did I avoid or resist interruptions?	
5. Did I remain connected to the patient while using my computer or other tech device?	
6. If family members were present, did I give them my full attention when they were talking?	

What one thing did I do especially well?

What one thing do I want to do differently to be even more effective?

🔍 Personal Spot-Check: On Using Technology with Patient

With this patient, how well did I combine use of a technology device with effective communication with the patient?	YES ✓
1. Did I log in and out in front of the patient, so the patient wouldn't worry about confidentiality?	
2. Did I alternate my attention between the patient and the device, instead of trying to multi-task?	
3. When I asked a question, did I look at the patient while he or she responded?	
4. If the patient was discussing a concern or emotional issue, did I keep my focus on the patient?	
5. Did I invite the patient to see what I was writing or reading?	

What one thing did I do especially well?

What one thing do I want to do differently to be even more effective?

Patient Feedback: On Mindful Practice

Dear Patient,
I'm asking you for feedback on how well I listen, so I can be a better doctor. Tell me, please: during our visit today, how well did I listen to you?

	YES ✓
1. Did I maintain eye contact with you while we were talking?	
2. Did I seem to be tuned in to what you were saying?	
3. Did I listen without interrupting?	
4. Did I avoid letting use of the computer or other device hurt our communication?	
5. Did I make you feel important?	

What do you suggest I do next time in order to improve my effectiveness? _____

_____

THANK YOU!

Family Feedback: On Mindful Practice

Dear Family Member,
I'm asking you for feedback, so I can be a better doctor. Tell me,
please: During our visit today, how well did I listen to you and
the patient?

	YES ✓
1. Did I maintain eye contact with you while we were talking?	
2. Did I maintain eye contact with the patient while we were talking?	
3. Did I seem to be listening well?	
4. Did I pay attention without interrupting?	
5. Did I avoid letting use of the computer or other tech device hurt my communication with you or your family member?	
6. Do you think I made the patient feel important?	
7. Did I make you feel important?	

What can I do in the future to be a more effective listener? _____

_____

THANK YOU!

Peer/Colleague Feedback: On Mindful Practice

Dear Colleague,
I'm working on listening more effectively and attentively to
my patients... being more mindful when I'm interacting with them.
Please help by observing my interaction and sharing your
perceptions and suggestions.

	YES ✓
1. Did I maintain eye contact with the patient when the patient was talking?	
2. Did I appear to be tuned in to what the patient was saying?	
3. Did I avoid interrupting?	
4. Did I avoid letting the computer or other tech device hurt my communication with the patient?	
5. Do you think I acted in a way that made the patient feel important?	
6. If family members were present, did I give them undivided attention when they were talking?	

What can I do in the future to be a more effective listener? _____

_____

What did I do particularly well? _____

THANK YOU!

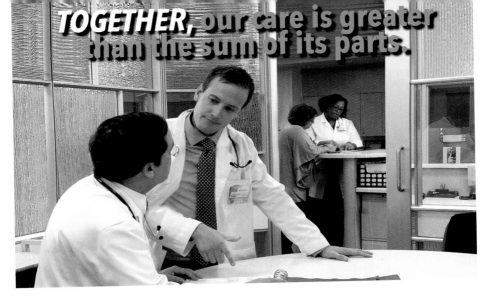

TOGETHER, our care is greater than the sum of its parts.

4. Collaboration and Teamwork

"The system of care is changing from an individual-based sport to a team-based sport."

Steven Weinberger, MD
Executive VP and CEO, American College of Physicians
Healthcare IT News, December 2, 2011

🔍 QUICK SELF-CHECK	YES ✓
1. Do I show leadership qualities in interactions with others on the care team?	
2. Do I acknowledge and appreciate coworkers who are involved in the patient's care?	
3. Do I open my mind to diverse perspectives?	
4. Do I connect and communicate with coworkers, so we will be on the same page with the patient's care?	
5. Do I communicate with empathy in strained interactions with colleagues?	
6. When I do a handoff to another member of the care team, do I build the patient/family's confidence in the next person down the line?	
7. Do I initiate relationship-building conversations with coworkers in order to ensure mutual understanding, harmony and cooperation?	
8. Do I act as a positive role model for collaboration and teamwork?	

Physicians who foster collaboration and teamwork can answer YES to these questions. These behaviors encourage colleagues and all members of the care team to contribute, cooperate and support you, each other and the patient.

The Emerging Role of the Physician

Due to the complexity of healthcare delivery and the many people involved in any one patient's care, the role of physician has shifted.

In **Academic Medicine**, Leape et al (2010) assert that healthcare has been organized around physician methods that favor physicians' "individual privilege and autonomy" as opposed to collaboration, teamwork and the inclusion of others in decisions. As a physician, YOU are team leader in a WEB of relationships with the patient and family at the center. The entire web of relationships is intended to promote the patient's well-being and full functioning. It used to be that physicians were captains of the ship responsible and accountable for all decisions, treatments and failures of the entire healthcare team. But this concept has lost favor.

Read an excerpt from one physician's blog about the "captain of the ship" concept.

"The captain of the ship is not one physician anymore! The captain is a collaboration of expert opinions, opinions that all of the physicians, nurses, and social workers, as well as the patient and their family bring to the table. If any one physician over-rides another without respectful communication or retreats from working out differences of opinion, it's bad for the team."

With team care now the standard, and the onset of care models like Accountable Care Organizations and the Patient-Centered Medical Home that require even more effective teamwork, the role of physician as "captain of the ship" is an anachronism. Physicians today need to act as team leaders and coaches in what are increasingly egalitarian, shared responsibility models.

 Facts!

According to the Institute for Healthcare Improvement, effective collaboration results in:

- Better coordination of patient care
- Improved compliance with core measures of safety, pain control and patient outcomes
- Shorter lengths of stay for inpatients
- Decreased emergency room use
- Fewer nursing home admissions following a hospital stay
- Decreased mortality one year after discharge
- Decreased overall health care costs
- And improved employee, physician AND patient satisfaction.

For care teams to be optimally effective, the people who comprise the team need to collaborate and respect each other's value and contributions.

Teamwork Breakdowns Are Consequential

Consider Jessie Gruman's Blog Entry:

> "It's difficult to imagine that professionals working in a practice or department or unit where they are constrained by their own colleagues' misbehavior are going to have the energy to invite us to learn about and share in decisions about our treatment; where preoccupation with hurt feelings and temper outbursts among staff will allow them to imagine what we must know and do to care for ourselves when we leave the hospital–and then help us plan how we'll do it…. We patients are insignificant bit players in an intense ongoing personal drama among those people who provide our care. We come and go, but the squabbles and turf battles and grudges among them spool out over years. Meanwhile, we can object directly, complain to administrators, change clinicians, or institutions to protect ourselves. And we can express our dissatisfaction in surveys and go public with our concerns on various rating sites, although our individual efforts will have little impact on a culture where disrespectful behavior by professionals is tolerated….
>
> Contemplate all this and then recall the clinicians who have listened to you and cared for you over the years. The ones who love their work and are committed to doing the best they can for each of us; the ones who work in settings where they are valued and respected and who bring energy and focus to their efforts to help us. A culture of respect in health care may be a very heavy lift in some places, but it already exists in practices and hospitals and clinics all over the country."

The Insidious Power of (d-i-s)-R-E-S-P-E-C-T.
Prepared Patient Forum; June 6th, 2012

With collaboration increasingly important, breakdowns in collaboration and teamwork become even more destructive. According to Zwarenstein and Reeves (2006), a growing empirical base suggests that failures of collaboration between professionals have a profound negative effect on health care and patient outcomes, "undermining the validity of clinical decisions, and interrupting or creating errors in the implementation of these decisions." The Joint Commission Sentinel Event Alert (Issue 40, 9/9/08) provides evidence that intimidating and disruptive behaviors on the part of physicians foster medical errors, contribute to poor patient satisfaction, foster preventable adverse outcomes, increase the cost of care, and cause excellent clinicians to seek other employment.

What kinds of collaboration breakdowns occur? No doubt, you've witnessed or experienced many firsthand–in both formal settings like interdisciplinary or multi-disciplinary meetings and in informal, backstage interactions like one-on-one conversations, emails, and phone calls.

- "I couldn't believe it. He called me into the room and in front of the patient, he said in an angry, accusing tone, 'Why hasn't her scan been scheduled?'"
- "He's an expert subspecialist and I've sent him a load of patients, but he doesn't get back to me when I call."
- "She screamed at me, 'How dare you bother me with this kind of question!'. Maybe her complaint was legit, but the WAY she talked to me? It was infuriating, and it does NOT make me want to help her."
- "I asked him if he had considered a different diagnosis, and he said, 'Well, well, well! When did YOU graduate from medical school?' He brings condescension to new heights."

Experiences like these discourage team members from supporting you and providing the best possible patient care.

⌕ Awareness Check *(Take a deep breath and be honest with yourself.)*

Common Breakdowns in Collaboration and Teamwork: Which have you experienced?	I have witnessed this	I have engaged in this
1. Reluctance or refusal to answer questions		
2. Not returning phone calls, pages, text or email messages		
3. Condescending language or voice tone		
4. Impatience with questions		
5. Bullying		
6. Disparaging remarks; slurs; putdowns; discouraging disagreement; public humiliation		
7. Claiming others' ideas as your own		
8. Angry outbursts; aggressive acts, like throwing instruments, charts or other things, pushing, grabbing, breaking things, banging the wall, pointing the finger, yelling, swearing		
9. Acts of unkindness, sabotage, divisiveness, infighting, scapegoating		

Common Breakdowns in Collaboration and Teamwork: Which have you experienced?	I have witnessed this	I have engaged in this
10. Belittling gestures e.g. deliberate eye-rolling, folding arms, staring into space when communication is attempted; body language aimed to discomfort the other		
11. Finding fault or nitpicking that goes beyond constructive professional feedback		
12. Ignoring, discounting or minimizing another's concerns		
13. So-called jokes and slurs based on race, ethnicity, religion, gender or sexual orientation		
14. 'Freezing out' or excluding others from participation in the work, social activities and informal conversation		
15. Devaluing people's roles, gender, and others different from yourself		
16. Expressing elitist attitudes about your education, experience and importance; a "better than" attitude		
17. Backbiting		
18. Passing judgment or censuring staff members in front of patients and families and other staff members		
19. Shaming others for negative outcomes		
20. Gratuitous negative comments about another physician's care		
21. Intimidating physical behavior such as a stiff posture, hitting or assault		
22. Creating rigid or inflexible barriers to requests for assistance or cooperation		

In contrast, coworkers thrive in an atmosphere of regard, compassion and respect.

- "Suzanne, you've been very important to Mrs. Baker's care. I know she and her family appreciate it."
- "Randy, you've established great rapport with the family. What's your thinking about what we can do to engage them in planning for Mr. Halstein's discharge."
- "No need to apologize for calling me so late, Sarita. I know you have our patient's best interest at heart."

Physician as Team Leader

Patients, families, your practice and care teams look to YOU to create a COMMUNITY of caring. When you ACT as team leader ---when you foster mutual respect and trust, everyone wins---you, your patients and the entire healthcare team.

As team leader, you have the power to:

- Set the tone
- Establish high standards
- Make sure people feel valued
- Publicly recognize contributions to the team and the patient
- Teach, give feedback and coach
- And express optimism and regard for the team

To help you maximize your central role as team leader, consider the following Six Rules of Thumb for inspiring cooperation and collaboration.

 Based on the Evidence: Skills for Collaboration and Teamwork

👍 Six Rules of Thumb: Effective Collaboration and Teamwork

1. Acknowledge and appreciate everyone involved in the patient's care.

2. Invite diverse perspectives and open your mind to them.

3. Communicate with empathy in strained interactions with coworkers.

4. Transfer trust during handoffs by speaking positively about the next person down the line.

5. Ask for what you need or want in a clear and caring way.

6. Initiate relationship-building conversations.

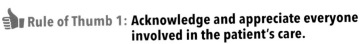 Rule of Thumb 1: **Acknowledge and appreciate everyone involved in the patient's care.**

In his breakthrough book, **The Checklist Manifesto: How to Get Things Right**, Atul Gewande demonstrates the power of simply acknowledging people on the care team. He found that, when all individuals on the team introduced themselves to each other before the surgery, the average number of complications and deaths dipped by 35 percent. Simple regard for each other's name encourages full participation to the benefit of the patient.

When you actively and frequently appreciate the people on your team, you use the power of acknowledgement even more.

- "Thanks for your help. I really appreciate it."
- "Raj, thanks for seeing Mrs. Albee so fast."
- "Mrs. Malloy, Helen is terrific. We're lucky to have her on our team."
- "Ms. Baxter raved about your care. I wanted you to know!"
- "That's a really good observation. How does that change what you think we should do?"

When you express appreciation and thanks, you receive support in return, and you foster a positive, appreciative climate that helps everyone do their best.

Rule of Thumb 2: **Invite diverse perspectives and open your mind to them.**

- "I told him I was worried about the patient going home so soon, and he said, "Where did you get YOUR medical degree?"
- "I'm the doctor. I'll decide that."

When physicians belittle or dismiss others' ideas, patients lose out on valuable perspectives and you lose respect and cooperation. Make it overtly clear that you value people's ideas.

- "What do you think, Helen? You've had a lot of experience with similar patients."
- "Mrs. Berger's daughter called and said we've been telling her different things. Let's talk so we can get on the same page, so she won't be confused."

Let's face it, none of us is as smart as all of us together. When you draw others into the dialogue, they feel valued and the patient benefits.

Rule of Thumb 3: **Communicate with empathy in strained interactions with coworkers.**

Most likely, others on the care team want to do a good job. They want to do their part. They want to be supportive. And they mean well. But so often, everyone is working under pressure with many patients to see, delays, challenges accessing results, calls to return, people making demands, paperwork, and so much more. The realities get in the way and can cause escalating stress that frustrates team members and produces exasperating, frustrating, less-than-admirable behavior. It doesn't help to enter into the cycle of negativity and frustration. What helps is to nip the frustrations in the bud by expressing empathy to coworkers and giving them the benefit of the doubt in strained interactions.

Imagine this: A patient complains that she's eager to go home. You've released the patient, but the nurse hasn't completed the discharge. And the family is complaining to you. In your frustration, you could say:

> *"What's holding up Mrs. Smith's discharge? I told her she could go home. Her family's on my case, and you're holding up the works!"*

No surprise, the nurse feels resentful. Now what if you were to include empathy in your message?

> *"I had told Mrs. Smith that she could go home today and her family is very eager to get her home. I realize you have a load of demands on you. Still, can you possibly finish her discharge now, so she can go home? I'll really appreciate it and I know Mrs. Smith and her family will too."*

With this more empathic approach, you would be much more likely to get the result you want.

By empathy, we mean acknowledging the coworker's feelings in an accepting, nonjudgmental way.

- "I realize you're under a lot of pressure!"
- "I'm sorry if this adds another pressure to your already hectic day."
- "It looks like this has been VERY frustrating for you today."
- "I value your ideas and appreciate your determination to do the right thing for our patient."
- "I know it's not easy to know what's happening with every patient every minute!"

Your use of empathy is especially important when you talk to a staff member who made a mistake or omission in caring for your patient. Now, your instinct might be to show anger. But if you respond with insults or anger, the true issue fades into the background. For the employee and others on the team, the issue becomes your behavior. And the next time you work with the same team, they'll worry not about how to do the right thing, but instead about whether you're going to act out again. When you're upset with a coworker, you'll be much more likely to get the performance you want if your approach is direct, empathic and respectful. For example, "James, I know you want to do the right thing for our patients. In this situation, you didn't check in on the patient as I requested, and the patient's problem with the medication went unnoticed, putting the patient at risk."

👍 Rule of Thumb 4: Transfer trust during handoffs by speaking positively about the next person down the line.

Think of the MANY handoffs you perform in a typical day. You hand off patients to hospitalists, to specialists, to your office manager, to a nurse, to an outpatient facility and more. The fact is, patients and their families become ANXIOUS during handoffs. While they might very well trust you, they don't know whether they'll be in good hands as they proceed to the next person or team down the line.

The success of a handoff depends greatly on your effective communication. You have the power to transfer the trust from you to your colleagues and help patients and families feel secure---by the words you use when you explain the handoff to the patient and their family.

- "I suggest you see Dr. Marks. She's a wonderful radiation oncologist and you'll find her both expert and very caring. You'll be in good hands with Dr. Marks."
- "Dr. Malkin will take over for me tonight. He's an excellent hospitalist and will stop in to see you for sure."
- "Ralph will walk you through the procedure. He is one of our finest techs and will make sure you're clear about it and comfortable while he's doing it."

Sometimes this is called "managing up". We think of it as an opportunity to "pay it forward." Also, colleagues will view you as a team player. Patients will view you as a leader who knows the capabilities and talents of everyone on your team. Also, when you express confidence in others on the care team, coworkers do their best work and they reciprocate with regard for you. The result: Patients and families benefit.

👍 Rule of Thumb 5: Ask for what you need or want in a clear and caring way.

Imagine this situation: You ask a coworker to follow-up with a patient's family, and he doesn't follow up in what you think is a timely fashion. You resent this.

There are many ways you could respond that would make matters worse, such as:
- You could do nothing and just stew with resentment.
- You could disparage the person to the patient, making it clear that this other person, not you, failed to follow through.

Before acting in any of these ways, ask yourself if you stated your request clearly and with caring in the first place. A clear, specific, forthright request enables the two of you to reach a shared understanding, resolving any issues before they arise.

> *"Max, I'm asking you to explain your recommendations to Mr. Johnson's family by 3 PM today, since I'm going to be meeting with them at around 4 o'clock. I'll really appreciate it."*

If you were not utterly clear initially, then it shouldn't be surprising that Max didn't follow up in what you thought was a timely fashion.

Another case in point involves asking nurses directly for what you need. It's not uncommon to hear physicians frustrated with calls from nurses that feel like they take too long. While physicians are trained to be very concise in transmitting information, many nurses have been trained to be more fully descriptive. The SBAR technique (Situation-Background-Assessment- Recommendation) developed by Michael Leonard at Kaiser Permanente has gained favor among physicians and nurses because it is an efficient framework for transmitting information that bridges communication styles. If you are not getting information in an efficient and effective way, come right out and respectfully ask your nurse colleagues to use the SBAR framework. Clarify your expectations and prevent frustrating interactions later on.

SBAR (Situation, Background, Assessment, Recommendation)

A technique for communicating critical information that requires immediate attention and action concerning a patient's condition

- **Situation** – What is going on with the patient? "I am calling about Mrs. Joseph in room 251. Chief complaint is shortness of breath of new onset."

- **Background** – What is the clinical background or context? "Patient is a 62-year-old female post-op day one from abdominal surgery. No prior history of cardiac or lung disease."

- **Assessment** – What do I think the problem is? "Breath sounds are decreased on the right side with acknowledgment of pain. Would like to rule out pneumothorax."

- **Recommendation** – What would I do to correct it? "I feel strongly the patient should be assessed now. Are you available to come in?"

Source: Institute for Healthcare Improvement. Guidelines for communicating with physicians using the SBAR process. http://www.ihi.org/IHI/Topics/PatientSafety / SafetyGeneral/ Tools/SBARTechniqueforCommunicationASituationalBriefing Model. htm. 2004

Or consider the STICC protocol used by the U.S. Forest Service. This protocol invites discussion and comes across as especially respectful.

STICC Protocol

- **Situation** – Here's what I think we face.

- **Task** – Here's what I think we should do.

- **Intent** – Here's why.

- **Concern** – Here's what we should keep our eye on.

- **Calibrate** – Talk to me. Tell me if you don't understand, can't do it, or see something I do not.

Source: JCAHO, The Joint Commission Guide to Improving Staff Communication. Oakbrook Terrace, IL: Joint Commission Resources; 2005.

Through respectful conversation, make your expectations clear. Listen to the other person's response. Work toward agreement on how you will proceed and you will prevent many frustrations and resentments down the road.

Just as family relationships need tending, so do work relationships. By asking for what you want clearly and forthrightly, you can SHAPE your relationships so they serve your patients and make YOUR work much more fulfilling.

Rule of Thumb 6: Initiate relationship-building conversations.

Give your team relationships a jumpstart. Initiate relationship-building conversations.

- "We're going to be working together a lot and I want a really good relationship with you. Can we take a few minutes and get to know each other?"
- "We're both under a lot of pressure. I'd like to talk with you about how we can help each other."

Relationship-building conversations like these take time upfront, but they SAVE time later by making your relationships more collaborative.

Wrap-Up

Given the complexity of patient care, of necessity, teams care for patients. Others on the care team rely on you to provide team leadership and oil the wheels for effective teamwork and collaboration. As role model and coach, you can have a powerful impact on the quality of life for the care team, on the experience of the patient and family and on your own sense of pride and fulfillment in your daily work.

Highlights for Review: Collaboration and Teamwork

Rules of Thumb	Examples
1. Acknowledge and appreciate everyone involved in the patient's care.	"Mrs. Baxter raved about your care. I wanted you to know!"
2. Invite diverse perspectives and open your mind to them.	"What do you think, Helen? You've had a lot of experience with similar patients."
3. Communicate with empathy in strained interactions with coworkers.	"I realize your plate is already full with the pressure of so many new patients at once."
4. Transfer trust during handoffs by speaking positively about the next person down the line.	"Ralph will walk you through the procedure. He's one of our finest techs and will make sure you're comfortable."
5. Ask for what you need or want in a clear and caring way.	"I'm asking you to tell me when you will be delayed, so I can adjust the patient's expectations."
6. Initiate relationship-building conversations.	"We're both under a lot of pressure. I'd like to talk with you about how we can help each other."

1. Cleary P D, A hospitalization from hell: A patient's perspective on quality. **Ann Intern Med**;2003;138(1):33–9.

2. Ellingson L, Communication, collaboration and teamwork among health care professionals. **Communication Research Trends**; Centre for the Study of Communication and Culture;V21 (2002) No. 3.

3. Fagin, C. (1992). "Collaboration between nurses and physicians: No longer a choice." **Academic Medicine**;67(5), 295-303.

4. Joint Commission, Behaviors that undermine a culture of safety. **Sentinel Event Alert**; 40:July 9, 2008.

5. Larson, E, The impact of physician-nurse interaction on patient care. **Holistic Nursing Practice**;1999:13(2), 38-46.

6. Leape L et al. Perspective: A culture of respect, part 1: The nature and causes of disrespectful behavior. **Acad Med;**2012;87:845-852.

7. Leape L et al., Perspective: A culture of respect, Part 2: Creating a culture of respect. **Acad Med**;22;May 2012.

8. LeTourneau B, Physicians and nurses: Friends or foes? **Journal of Healthcare Management**; 2004:49(1), 12-14.

9. Lindeke, L et al., Nurse-physician workplace collaboration. **OJIN: The Online Journal of Issues in Nursing;** Vol. 10 No. 1, Manuscript 4.

10. Nairl DM et al., Frequency of nurse–physician collaborative behaviors in an acute care hospital. **J Interprofessional Care**; 2011;1–6.

11. Pronovost P et al., Improving communication in the ICU using daily goals. **J Crit Care**;2003;18(2):71–5.

12. Van Norman G, Interdisciplinary team issues. **Ethics in Medicine**; University of Washington, April 11, 2008.

13. Zwarenstein, M and Reeves S, Working together but apart: Barriers and routes to nurse-physician collaboration. **The Joint Commission**;2002:28(5), 242-247.

14. Zwarenstein M & Reeves S, Knowledge translation and interprofessional collaboration: Where the rubber of evidence-based care hits the road of teamwork. **Journal of Continuing Education in the Health Professions**; 2006:26,46–54.

15. Zwarenstein M et al., Interprofessional collaboration: Effects of practice-based interventions on professional practice and healthcare outcomes. **Cochrane Database of Systematic Reviews 2009**; Issue 3; No CD000072.

- Personal Spot Check
- Patient Feedback
- Family Feedback
- Peer/Colleague Feedback

Personal Spot-Check: Collaboration and Teamwork

In this team situation, which best practices did I use?	YES ✓
1. I acknowledged and appreciated my coworkers.	
2. I welcomed different viewpoints.	
3. I communicated with every coworker in a respectful way.	
4. I spoke positively about my coworkers to patients, their family members and/or other coworkers.	
5. Before this encounter, I communicated with others involved in the patient's care, so we could be on the same page with the patient.	
6. I acted as a positive role model for collaboration and teamwork.	

What strengths did I demonstrate as I worked collaboratively with my coworkers?

What could I have done better or differently to foster respect, inclusion and teamwork?

Dear Patient,
A team of people have been involved in your care. All of us on the
team want to collaborate and communicate well with one another
for your sake. To be an effective member of your care team, I'm asking
you for feedback about how I behaved with my coworkers.
I'll greatly appreciate it.

	YES ✓
1. Have you seen me acknowledge and appreciate my coworkers?	
2. Do I seem to welcome different viewpoints?	
3. Do I seem to communicate with my coworkers in a respectful way?	
4. Have I spoken positively about my coworkers to you?	
5. Do you feel that the various people involved in your care are communicating well with each other?	
6. Do you think I act as a positive role model for collaboration and teamwork?	

When have you wished people on your care team were communicating with one another more effectively? _____

_____

Please suggest one thing I can do in the future to be more effective. _____

_____

Other comments, wishes, suggestions or concerns? _____

_____

_____

THANK YOU!

Dear Family Member,
A team of people have been involved in the patient's care.
All of us on the team want to collaborate and communicate
well with one another for the good of patients and families.
So I can be an effective member of the care team, I'm asking you
for feedback about how you saw me behave in team situations.
I'll greatly appreciate it.

	YES ✓
1. Have you seen me acknowledge and appreciate coworkers?	
2. Have you seen me welcome different views?	
3. Do I communicate in a respectful way with my coworkers?	
4. Have I spoken positively about my coworkers in front of you?	
5. Do the people involved in the patient's care seem to communicate well with each other?	
6. Do you think I act as a positive role model for collaboration and teamwork?	

When have you wished people on our care team had communicated with one another
more effectively? _____

_____

Please suggest one thing I can do in the future to be more effective. _____

_____

Other comments, wishes, suggestions or concerns? _____

_____

THANK YOU!

Dear Colleague,
I want to be an effective team member who collaborates well and
supports others on our care team for the sake of the patient and
the team's morale and effectiveness. Please give me feedback about
how well I demonstrate teamwork and collaboration.

	YES ✓
1. Do I seem to acknowledge and appreciate colleagues involved in the patient's care?	
2. Do you think I welcome diverse perspectives?	
3. Do I communicate with you in a respectful way?	
4. When I hand off a patient or a patient's information to you, do I do so in a way that eases your way with the patient?	
5. Do I make myself available when you and I need to discuss a patient's condition or care plan?	
6. Do you think I do my part in making sure you and I are on the same page regarding the patient's care?	
7. Do you see me as a positive role model for collaboration and teamwork?	

What situation comes to mind when you wish I had behaved differently in order to work well with you or others on the team, for the sake of the patient? _____

_____

Other feedback or suggestions? _____

_____

_____

THANK YOU!

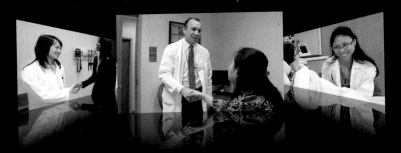

In each encounter, from the very beginning to the very end, stay engaged.

Help patients and families feel:
• *Welcome* • *Respected* • *Cared About* • *Heard*

5. Effective Openings and Closings

🔍 QUICK SELF-CHECK	YES ✓
1. Do I greet my patients warmly?	
2. If there are family members present, do I welcome them and introduce myself?	
3. Do I call my patients by name--the name they prefer?	
4. Do I connect with the patient immediately by showing knowledge of the patient?	
5. Do I encourage the patient to describe all concerns before I dive into any one, so we can set a manageable agenda together?	
6. If there are family members present, do I ask them to share their hopes for the visit as well?	
7. Do I check the patient's (and family member's) understanding and comfort with next steps before ending the visit?	
8. Do I make it clear that the visit is ending and make an effort to help the patient (and family member) feel closure?	
9. Do I say goodbye warmly, remaining mindful with the patient and wishing the patient well?	
10. Do I make the last six seconds of our interaction a positive memory?	

Are you deliberate about your behavior during openings and closings, since these are powerful, influential touchpoints in the patient experience?

Every day, with every patient, family member and coworker, in every single encounter, you engage in an opening and a closing, whether you do so consciously or not. How you execute your openings and closings has a great impact on:

- Patient and family trust and confidence in you
- Patient and family anxiety, engagement and openness
- Comprehension of information, and
- Commitment to the plan of care and follow-through

Because patient-centered openings and closings contribute to positive outcomes and high patient ratings of your communication quality, it's likely that, by rethinking and becoming more deliberate in your approaches, you can achieve an even more positive impact.

> - **Openings:** How you greet the patient and family, build rapport, engage the patient and family, and focus the encounter
>
> - **Closings:** How you end the encounter so that the patient and family members feel safe, cared for, confident, committed, clear about their next steps, and positive about you and their experience

 Based on the Evidence: The Elements of an Effective Opening

How can you make your opening effective every time?

✋ Five Rules of Thumb: Effective Openings

1. Before entering, prepare.

2. Enter and make the most of your first six seconds.

3. Personalize your care by showing knowledge of the patient.

4. Elicit all of the patient's (and family member's) concerns.

5. Together, negotiate the agenda.

In the first few moments, you create a powerful first impression that can color the entire encounter.

Rule of Thumb 1: **Before entering, prepare.**

Early on in the visit, it's important to show knowledge of the patient-- to immediately recognize the patient as an individual.

Before entering:

- Scan the patient's medical history.
- Identify visits with other providers and any follow-up tests and results.
- Be ready with a comment that shows two kinds of knowledge of the patient: something personal and something about the person's medical history.
- Take a deep breath and become fully present.
- Knock and wait three seconds before entering.

 ### Rule of Thumb 2: **Enter and make the most of your first six seconds.**

Set the tone for the visit by making your first impression very positive.

- Make eye contact and say hello.
- Greet the patient by name.
- Introduce yourself and your role to both the patient and the family.
- Approach the patient.
- Ask permission to sit and turn off distracting noises.
- Sit down and lean in.
- Be consciously and intentionally mindful in your words and nonverbal behavior.

Note: Getting the patient's name right is very important to patients. Initially, use a salutation and the patient's last name. Then, ask the patient what they PREFER to be called. Note it and make a point of calling the patient by their preferred name from then on. Use the patient's name often. **And be sure to avoid words like** "Honey, Sweetheart, and Dear," since more than 60% of patients find these well-intended words disrespectful.

 ### Rule of Thumb 3: **Personalize your care by showing knowledge of the patient.**

Right after greeting the patient and settling into an attentive posture:

Demonstrate Two Kinds of Knowledge	Examples
Personal Knowledge	• *"Good morning, Mr. Schmidt. Do I remember right that you went to Florida for vacation right after I saw you last?"* • *"I hear your grandkids were in to see you last night! They doted on you, I hope!"*
Medical Knowledge	• *"I hear you had some pain during the night. How's your pain now?"* • *"Last time you were here, you had a hacking cough. How is that now?"*

If you didn't have a chance to prepare, ask, *"Would you give me a moment to refresh my memory?"* Then, take a minute to tune in to THIS patient's information.

👍 Rule of Thumb 4: Elicit all patient (and family) concerns, and add your own.

After your greeting and establishing rapport, elicit all concerns. Listen and don't interrupt. Then, because the patient's first concern is often not the most important, encourage the patient to express all of their concerns by asking, "What else? What else is concerning you?" If you're aware of all of the patient's concerns upfront, you can create a do-able agenda for the encounter and prevent those maddening hand-on-doorknob questions.

Jot down the patient's (and family's) concerns as the patient walks you through them, so you can refer to your list when you proceed to set the agenda together. Also, add any concerns that you want to address with the patient. Especially in medical visits, these might include chronic care and preventive health issues that are medically indicated.

- **Physician:** "So, it's been two days since your surgery. How you are you feeling today?"
- **Patient:** "Not great."
- **Physician:** "Tell me all of your concerns and then we can work our way through the ones that are most important to talk about today."
- **Patient:** "I was nauseous all night and I know I need to eat to get healthy."
- **Physician:** "Well, let's get that nausea under control so you can eat and get stronger. Tell me about your pain too, so we can manage both problems better."
- **Patient:** "I think the pain medicine is causing the nausea, but my pain isn't bad right now."
- **Physician:** "OK, that helps a lot. And what else is on your mind today–any other concerns."
- **Patient:** "My back hurts."
- **Physician:** "I'm sorry to hear that. OK. Anything else?"
- **Patient:** "I want to discuss whether I should do my other knee sooner or later."
- **Physician:** "OK. Noted! Did we miss anything?
- **Patient:** "That's all."
- **Physician:** "Great! And there are a couple of things I'd like to talk with you about: What you'll need to do to prevent infection once you get home and when it makes sense to go home. Now let's figure out which of your concerns and mine we want to address today for sure. Then, if we can't do a good job on the other concerns in the time we have, we can arrange another time. How does that sound to you?"
- **Patient:** "Okay."

Now, you might think you don't have time to listen to the patient's whole story, ask "what else" and encourage the patient to speak freely. Research has shown that, while this takes between one and two more minutes upfront, you save time overall because you can negotiate an agenda that fully address the patient's main priorities and avoid pressing doorknob questions.

Rule of Thumb 5: Together, negotiate the agenda.

Then, with ALL of the patients' concerns in hand, work TOGETHER to create the visit agenda, assuring the patient that less urgent concerns will be addressed at another time.

Together, negotiate the agenda: The Specifics
- Don't do a diagnostic dive until you establish the agenda together.
- Order the issues by medical urgency and the patient's level of distress.
- Discuss a priority order with the patient.
- Together: Agree on an agenda that fits your time constraints.
- Use partnership language: "We", "us" and "together"

- **Physician:** "So, we have a lot to discuss. You want help with your nausea, your knee pain and your back pain. And you want to discuss when to do your other knee. I want to be sure we discuss your home care and also when you can plan on going home. This is a lot. I'd like to agree on the priorities with you, and not try to handle all of it in this one conversation."
- **Patient:** "Well, I'm really bothered by the pain."
- **Physician:** "I'm so sorry. Let's definitely start with your discomfort---your knee and back pain and your nausea. I really want you to be comfortable."
- **Patient:** "Okay."
- **Physician:** "And I'd really like to begin talking about our plan for your going home."
- **Patient:** "Okay. Me too."
- **Physician:** "And how about if we postpone talking about doing your other knee until an office visit after you're home?"
- **Patient:** "Okay."
- **Physician:** "Great! So, let's address your pain and nausea first."
- **Patient:** "Good."

Important: By setting the agenda together, you both have a stake in it and you establish the concept of time limits upfront. By making the patient's main concerns top priority, you're sure to address these, so patients will be more likely to feel satisfied with the encounter. And you can clarify which agenda items will need to be postponed to another visit.

So, you've welcomed the patient and family, built rapport, showed knowledge of the patient, listened to the patient tell their story, elicited all concerns, added your own, and then together, negotiated a manageable visit agenda. That's an effective opening.

 Based on the Evidence: The Elements of an Effective Closing

How you close an encounter affects the patient's (and family's) feelings about the encounter as well. After all, your endings leave patients with a memory that leaves along with them. Also, how you close the encounter affects:

- The patient's grasp of and adherence to the care plan
- The patient's assessment of the experience that they will share on surveys and with family and friends
- The patient's likelihood of returning to and recommending you to others

Three Closings That Don't Work

	Example
1. The physician is so focused on the tasks and plan that he or she does not actually bring the encounter to a conscious close.	**Patient:** "No, I don't have any more questions right now." **Physician:** "OK, I'll prepare that prescription for you and you can pick it up on your way out." **The patient** doesn't realize that the physician is finished and the patient waits. The patient feels unfinished, forgotten, and a bit disregarded. The patient leaves with a negative feeling.
2. The physician detaches prematurely, with no more than an abrupt goodbye.	**Physician:** "So, that's it for today. Any other questions before we end? OK, it was good seeing you and I hope you feel better soon." **The physician** immediately turns away and starts entering progress notes in the computer. Feeling awkward, the patient eventually leaves. The patient concludes that the physician couldn't wait to get away from them.
3. The physician is finished, but the patient isn't. The physician has mentally moved on. The patient feels unfinished, rushed and irritated.	**Mrs. Harris** still speaking: "And I'm really starting to get depressed." **The physician** walks to door and with hand on door says, "Sorry, Mrs. Harris. I must move on. Our time is up. I'll stop by tomorrow and we can talk further." **Patient:** "Okay."

The Effective Close

The *last impression* you make leaves a *lasting impression*. Be sure that your closing accomplishes these three purposes:

- The patient and family understand next steps and are comfortable with and committed to them.
- Everyone feels closure.
- The patient leaves with a positive memory of you and the encounter.

👍 Three Rules of Thumb: Effective Closings

1. Check the patient's and family member's understanding and comfort with next steps.

2. Ensure closure.

3. Make the last 6 seconds a positive memory.

Rule of Thumb 1: Check the patient's and family member's understanding and comfort with next steps.

Use the tried-and-true "teach back" technique.	• *"So, I want to make sure we did a good job of coming up with a clear plan. Tell me what you understand to be the next steps?"* • *"So, let's review our discussion to make sure we're on the same page."* • *"I know your daughter will ask you about our visit today. What will you tell her?"*

Rule of Thumb 2: Ensure closure.

Make it very clear that the visit is nearing an end and do all you can to help the patient feel finished. Help the patient and family leave with clarity and a sense of security, and it will prevent phone calls later.	• *"Is there one last question you have before we end?"* • *"I look forward to seeing you tomorrow, and we'll keep working to get all your concerns addressed. Can everything else wait until then?"* • *"So I think we've addressed our agenda for today. Are you feeling finished? How did we do in addressing your priority concerns?"*

Rule of Thumb 3: Make the last six seconds a positive memory.

After achieving closure, make sure the last six seconds create a positive last (and lasting) impression.

Stay mindful–attentive to the patient until the very last moment.

Offer good wishes and a warm goodbye.

Physician: "It was good seeing you, Susan, and I hope you feel better soon. Don't hesitate to call if you have a problem. And please give my regards to your mother."

Susan: "OK, thanks!"

The physician walks Susan to the door, staying totally present to her as she begins walking down the hall, or, better yet, the physician walks Susan to the front.

And Please Note!

Just after the visit ends, make a habit of adding a sticky note to the patient's chart to remind you of personal info you can use in your next encounter to reconnect with the patient. Most health records have a sticky note function and this reduces the demands on your memory!

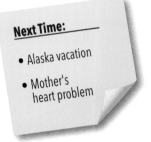

Next Time: _____

• Alaska vacation

• Mother's heart problem

Wrap-Up

Your behaviors during the beginning and end of an encounter have a disproportionately great impact on patients' feelings about their experience. By fine-tuning your opening and closing routines, you will be perceived as the caring physician you are.

👍 Rules of Thumb: The Effective Opening

1. Before entering, prepare.	• Scan the patient's medical history, visits with other doctors and test results. • Prepare comments that show personal & medical knowledge of patient. • Take a deep breath and become fully present. • Knock and wait three seconds before entering.
2. Enter and make the most of your first six seconds.	• Make eye contact and say hello to the patient (and their family). • Greet the patient by name. • Introduce yourself and your role. • Approach the patient, ask permission to sit. • Sit and lean in.
3. Personalize your care by showing your knowledge of the patient.	• Show personal knowledge. • Show medical knowledge.
4. Elicit and note all patient (and family) concerns, and add your own.	• First, listen for a full minute without interrupting. • Encourage the expression of all concerns: Ask, "What else?" • Add your own concerns.
5. Together, negotiate the visit agenda. *No diagnostic dive before agreeing on agenda.*	• Order issues by medical urgency and patient's level of distress. • Discuss priority order with the patient. • *Together:* Agree on an agenda that fits your time constraints. • Use partnership language: "We", "us" and "together."

Rules of Thumb: The Effective Closing

1. Check patient (and family) understanding and comfort with next steps.	• Use the tried-and-true "teach back" technique.
2. Ensure closure.	• "Is there one last question you have before we end?" • "So I think we've addressed our agenda for today. Are you feeling finished? How did we do in addressing your priority concerns?"
3. Make the last 6 seconds a positive memory.	• Stay mindful–attentive to the patient until the very last moment • Offer good wishes and a warm goodbye.

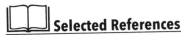 **Selected References**

1. Bakic NM, Successful doctor-patient communication and rapport-building as the key skills of medical practice. **Medicine and Biology**;2008;(15)2:74 – 79.

2. Frankel R and Stein T, Getting the most out of the clinical encounter: The Four Habits model. **The Permanente Journal**;Fall 1999;3:3.

3. Halpern J, Gathering the patient's story and clinical empathy. **The Permanente Journal**;Winter 2012:16:1.

4. Ness DE et al., Language and connectedness in the medical and psychiatric interview. **Patient Educ & Couns**;2007;68(2):139-144.

5. Robinson JD, Closing medical encounters: Two physician practices and their implications for the expression of patients' unstated concerns. **Social Science & Medicine**;53;2001:639-656.

6. Roter DL, Communication patterns in the primary care interview. 1997; **JAMA**; 277(4):350-6.

7. Scannell D, Narrative medicine: A case of baffling fatigue with a spectral twist; **Permanente Journal**;Winter 2012:Vol. 16, No. 1.

8. Stein TS and Kwan J, Thriving in a busy practice: Physician-patient communication training. **Eff Clin Pract**;1999;2(2):63-70.

Self-Improvement Tools: On Effective Openings and Closings

- **Personal Spot Check: Effective Openings**

- **Personal Spot Check: Effective Closings**

- **Patient Feedback**

- **Family Feedback**

- **Peer/Colleague Feedback**

🔍 Personal Spot-Check: Effective Openings

With this patient and family, which best practices did I use during my opening?	YES ✓
1. Did I prepare by collecting myself and familiarizing myself with the patient's record before entering the encounter?	
2. Did I greet the patient (and family) warmly?	
3. Did I call the patient by name?	
4. Did I connect with the patient immediately by showing knowledge of the patient?	
5. Did I elicit ALL patient (and family) concerns before setting an agenda with them?	
6. Did I listen without interrupting as the patient told their story?	

In my opening, what one thing did I do especially well?

What one thing do I want to do differently to be more effective?

🔍 Personal Spot-Check: Effective Closings

With this patient and family, which best practices did I use during my closing?	YES ✓
1. Did I check patient (and family) understanding and comfort with next steps before ending the visit?	
2. Did I invite one last question?	
3. Did I make it clear that the visit was ending and make an effort to help the patient (and family) feel closure?	
4. Did I say goodbye warmly?	
5. Did I stay totally focused on the patient (and family) until after our goodbye?	
6. Did I make the last six seconds of our interaction a positive memory?	

In my closing, what one thing did I do especially well?

What one thing do I want to do differently to be more effective?

Invite your patients to give you feedback.

- Early in an encounter, explain to the patient that you want to fine-tune your communication with your patients, and that you are currently focusing on how you open and close each visit. Ask them to notice how you open and close the visit, so they can provide you with brief written feedback afterward.

- Then, at the end of the encounter, invite your patient to complete a short report card. Thank them for their feedback and for helping you be a better doctor.

Dear Patient,
I'm asking you for feedback, so I can be a better doctor. Please tell me:
During our visit today, what did you think of how I greeted you and
opened our conversation?

	YES ✓
1. Did I greet you warmly?	
2. Did I call you by name---the name you prefer?	
3. Did I connect with you by showing knowledge of you and your medical history?	
4. Did I ask you to tell me all of your concerns before setting an agenda with you?	
5. Did you feel we worked together to set the agenda for the visit?	
6. Did we address the concerns you most wanted to discuss in today's visit?	
7. Before ending, did I check your understanding and comfort with next steps?	
8. Did I stay totally focused on you until after our goodbye?	
9. Did I make the last six seconds a positive memory for you?	
10. If family members were with you, did I welcome and engage with them in a positive way?	

What one thing did I do especially well? _____

_____

_____

What one thing do you suggest I do differently to be more effective? _____

_____

_____

THANK YOU!

Dear Family Member,
I'm asking you for feedback, so I can be a better doctor. Please tell me:
During my visit with the patient (and/or you) today, how effective was
I in the way I opened and closed the visit.

	YES ✓
1. Did I greet you warmly and introduce myself?	
2. Did I connect with the patient by showing personal knowledge of them and their medical history?	
3. Did I encourage the patient to state all of their concerns before setting an agenda for the visit?	
4. Did I ask you what YOU hoped to learn from the visit?	
5. Did you feel we worked together to set the agenda for the visit?	
6. Did we address the concerns you most wanted to discuss?	
7. Before ending, did I check the patient's and/or your understanding and comfort with next steps?	
8. Did I stay totally focused on you and the patient until after our goodbye?	
9. Did I make the last six seconds of our interaction a positive memory for you?	

What one thing did I do especially well? _____

_____

_____

What one thing do you suggest I do differently to be more effective? _____

_____

_____

THANK YOU!

Peer/Colleague Feedback: On Effective Openings and Closings

1. Learn from your colleagues. Notice how your colleagues handle openings and closings with patients and families. Consciously consider which elements make these important moments effective.

2. Invite a trusted colleague to observe you and give you feedback. You can use the following form to inquire.

Dear Colleague,
I'm asking you for feedback, so I can be a better doctor. When you were observing me with my patient (and family member), which best practices did you see me do?

	YES ✓
1. Did I greet the patient warmly and by name?	
2. If family members were present, did I make a point of greeting them warmly and introducing myself?	
3. Did I connect with the patient by showing knowledge of them as a person and knowledge of their medical history?	
4. Did I ask the patient to identify ALL of their concerns before setting an agenda?	
5. If family members were present, did I ask them what they hoped to learn from the visit?	
6. Did we work together to set the agenda for the visit?	
7. Did I address the concerns that mattered most to the patient (and family)?	
8. Before ending, did I check understanding and comfort with next steps?	
9. Did I stay totally focused on the patient (and family) until after our goodbye?	
10. Did I make the last six seconds a positive memory for the patient?	

What did I do especially well? _____

_____

_____

What are your suggestions? _____

_____

_____

THANK YOU!

Do nothing about me without me.

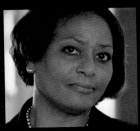 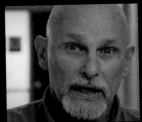 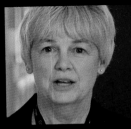

Treat me with dignity, respect and caring. Listen to me. Inform me. Involve my family. Partner in decisions about my care.

6. Engaging Patients and Families as Partners

🔍 QUICK SELF-CHECK	YES ✓
1. Do I encourage the patient to speak freely about their concerns before I intervene?	
2. Do I negotiate the visit agenda with the patient, instead of setting it myself?	
3. Do I invite the patient's ideas and viewpoints before making suggestions?	
4. Do I jointly discuss the patient's values and their impact on care options and decisions?	
5. Do I make a concerted effort to engage the patient in decisions about their care?	
6. When family members are present, do I invite their questions and address their concerns?	
7. If family members are present, do I involve them in decisions --with patient permission?	

If you answered YES to each of the above questions, you demonstrate behavior consistent with patient and family-centered care – behavior that encourages patients and their family members to engage with you and participate in decision-making.

Patient-centered care is a philosophy of care that encourages sharing with patients-- sharing decisions about your approach to the conversation and sharing decisions about care interventions and ongoing care. It also encourages caring for the whole person in context (not as a body part or disease) and considering personal preferences throughout the care process.

The shared decision making model:

- Recognizes that there are complex trade-offs in decisions about medical care
- Fulfills our ethical responsibility to inform patients fully about risks and benefits
- Ensures prominence of patients' values and preferences

In a patient-physician partnership, the physician:

- Tries to understand the person behind the disease (their health beliefs, concerns and expectations)
- Involves the family as much as the patient wants
- Asks open-ended questions
- Negotiates the agenda with the patient
- Addresses not only biomedical issues but also psychosocial issues.
- Shares information freely
- Explores the patient's values and preferences with the patient
- Shares decision-making
- Serves as *advisor* to the patient's goals and decisions

Dr. Rotering shares this reflection:

I remember as a much younger physician desperately and earnestly attempting to convince an aging gentleman with chronic heart disease to follow my strong medical recommendation to undergo an invasive procedure. His contrary opinion was equally strong despite his understanding of the value of this procedure. He simply no longer chose to agree to invasive procedures, for reasons he shared with me. He finally just reached over, patted my hand, and said, 'You know, Doc, there are worse things that can happen to you than dying.' I realized I had been unable to hear his voice or his choice above my righteous conviction that I knew what the BEST course was, and if there was a best course, that he (and all patients) should choose it!" He remains one of my greatest teachers.

Some physicians think that patient engagement is an either-or situation—that either they give their recommendation or they turn the decision-making over to the patient. It is not an either-or situation. It's a both/and situation. When there is a clearly preferred option based on evidence, it is important to advocate for this, recognizing that the decision itself belongs to the patient. When there are multiple options, it is our job to spend the time with the patient to surface their values and help them match the option that fits best with what they're looking to accomplish.

Consider the typical medical exam. It usually includes these steps:

- The greeting
- The patient's opening statement
- The history and physical
- The diagnosis
- The treatment
- And the closing

The only step at which the physician invites the patient to speak freely is during the patient's opening, when the physician wants to know the reason for the patient's visit. And even then, studies show that physicians interrupt the patient within 20 seconds.

These days, the vast majority of patients want to be involved in their care. They want to actively partner with their physicians when making decisions. And this is a promising trend, because patient engagement is related to optimal outcomes. Active patient involvement improves patient acceptance and adherence to physician recommendations and improves self-management of chronic conditions. In turn, this leads to improved physical functioning in everyday activities. (Lewin et al., 2001)

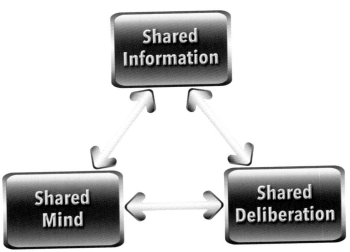

Empowerment, patient engagement, partnership, shared decision-making, activation---whatever you choose to call it, when patients are actively involved in their health care, they engage in:

- Healthier behaviors
- More effective self-monitoring
- And greater adherence to their care plan

The result: Better clinical results, and engaged patients rate physicians who engage them more highly than they rate physicians who don't.

Also, partnering with your patients makes you more effective, since you and the patient bring complementary areas of expertise to the encounter.

Physician is Expert on:	Patient is Expert on:
Diagnoses	Symptoms
Diseases	Goals and priorities
Treatments and remedies	Feelings and concerns
What ifs	Tradition, culture and values
Medical resources	Personal resources

To achieve the best possible care plan and outcomes, the two of you need to share your complementary expertise and work together.

How does partnering with patients and families look?

The CG-CAHPS Survey now includes a Supplemental Item Set on Shared Decision-Making. Providers focused on Patient-Centered Care are opting to include these items in their surveys:

- Provider talked about the reasons you might want to take a prescription medicine.
- Provider talked about the reasons you might not want to take a prescription medicine.
- When talking about starting or stopping a prescription medicine, provider asked you what was best for you.
- Provider talked about the reasons you might want to have surgery or procedure.
- Provider talked about the reasons you might not want to have surgery or procedure.
- When talking about surgery or procedure, provider asked you what was best for you.
- Provider talked about including family or friends in making health decisions.
- Provider talked about how much of your personal health information you wanted to share with family or friends.
- Provider respected your wishes about sharing personal health information with family or friends.
- You brought a family member or friend with you to talk with this provider.

The bottom line: When patient and family-centered care is in practice, a fly on the wall would see:

- A mutually respectful relationship
- Open, two-way communication
- Joint problem-solving and decision-making
- A concerted effort on your part to involve the patient's family members
- All in an atmosphere of psychological safety... warmth, collaboration and respect

"Yes, but...."

Some physicians think patients don't WANT to partner in their own care. Consider this Surgeon's Blog entry. "My patients tell me in so many words that they expect ME to make the decision (and to explain it to them, of course). If I were to do the whole "Here are your choices, you decide" tap dance demanded by the shared decision making paradigm, not only would I be doing these patients a disservice, but I'd annoy the heck out of them."

It's all too easy to take the reins when patients resist engagement, but it has quality consequences. If the patient doesn't WANT to be involved, of course, you can't force it. And it's respectful to honor their wishes. But because of the positive relationship between involvement and outcomes, assume they WANT involvement and TRY to engage them.

- "How would you like to PARTICIPATE in your care?"
- "How might you and I work TOGETHER to solve this?
- "I see you've been downloading information from the internet. Tell me what you've come up with so far, and I'll share my thoughts with you if you'd like."

The fact is: Most patients willingly participate in their care planning, even when they face complicated and difficult decisions.

2. Based on the Evidence: Skills for Engaging Patients and Families as Partners

Six Rules of Thumb: Engaging Patients and Families As Partners

1. Encourage the patient and family to speak up.

2. Share responsibility for the direction of the discussion.

3. Find out the patient's views and theories.

4. Use the language of partnership.

5. Collaborate on goal-setting and decision-making.

6. Involve the patient's family throughout the process.

Rule of Thumb 1: Encourage the patient and family to speak up.

Some patients have an engrained habit of passivity in the face of physician information and advice. Many need encouragement to speak up and participate.

- "I want you to ask me questions –ANY questions–about what you can expect, about anything I'm saying, about anything that isn't clear as we're talking. Please don't hesitate. We're working together on this!"
- "Tell me more. This is really helpful!" "
- And in cross-cultural situations: "I don't know your culture very well and I want to be respectful. Please help me understand."

Tips
- Invite their thinking, their feelings, their concerns and personal information about their lifestyle.
- Listen with respect. Be open to their ideas and concerns.
- Focus on the potential value of what the person is saying.
- ENCOURAGE the patient by finding something to validate.
- And talk in a nonjudgmental, positive tone.

 Rule of Thumb 2: Share responsibility for the discussion.

Feeling powerless is common to the patient experience. Yet, patients with their family members' support have the ultimate responsibility for implementing health decisions. You can ease patients' sense of powerlessness and also strengthen the patient's commitment to implement their decisions by sharing responsibility with them---by inviting them into the dialogue and giving them choices and the power to make them.

- **Acknowledge areas of agreement and disagreement**. "So, I'm suggesting that you go ahead with the surgery because it has a very low risk of side effects and will ease your pain. You're very hesitant about the surgery because of your past history."
- **Acknowledge that power is shared and validate patient's autonomy, sometimes deferring to the patient's wishes over your own**. "If you don't want us to do this, we won't."
- **Negotiate about discussions and choices**. "For your pain, you have some options here. You can take pain medicine that will relieve the pain, but it will make you sleepy and it will probably be hard to concentrate. Or you could tough it out which will be uncomfortable and draining. Or you could try some alternatives like acupuncture or massage. How are you thinking you would like to proceed?"

By sharing responsibility, your patients will engage with you, reflect on their options, and advocate on their own behalf.

👍 Rule of Thumb 3: **Find out the patient's (and their family members') views and theories.**

Before suggesting a care plan with the patient, find out their views and theories, as well as those of involved family members. That way, together, you can build a care plan that works for them. Invite their knowledge of complementary therapies in a nonjudgmental way. Listen with thoughtful consideration.

The Kleinman Questions are very helpful in asking the patient about their health-related beliefs. By asking these questions, you will understand the patient's perspective, be better able to address their needs together, and achieve their commitment to their care plan. Have these questions on hand to prompt yourself to use them to learn more about the patient's beliefs.

The Kleinman Questions

1. What do you think caused the problem?
2. Why do you think it happened when it did?
3. What do you think your sickness does to you? How does it work?
4. How severe is your sickness? Will it have a short course?
5. What kind of treatment do you think you should receive?
6. What are the most important results you hope to receive from this treatment?
7. What are the chief problems your sickness has caused for you?
8. What do you fear most about your sickness?

Kleinman, A., Eisenberg, L., & Good, B. (1978). Culture, illness, and care: Clinical lessons from anthropologic and cross-cultural research. *Annals of Internal Medicine*; 88(2), 251-258.

Three of the eight Kleinman questions are especially helpful with culturally diverse patients:

- What do YOU think caused the problem?
- What kind of TREATMENT do you think you should receive?
- What are the chief problems your sickness has CAUSED for you?

👍 Rule of Thumb 4: **Use the language of partnership.**

To encourage patient and family engagement and participation, use words like "we", "us", and "together" that make your intention to work together clear.

- "We're going to get to the bottom of this together."
- "I'm going to be with you every step of the way."
- "Let's figure out what's wrong, so we can help you feel better as soon as possible."

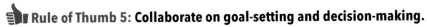 **Rule of Thumb 5: Collaborate on goal-setting and decision-making.**

For most clinical decisions, there are several reasonable management options. Surgery? Medicine? Watchful waiting? The options vary in their therapeutic and side effects. Unilateral or paternalistic decision-making disregards the patient's preferences. Preference-sensitive decisions require shared decision-making--a consensual process of reaching agreement about how to proceed.

To collaborate on decisions, the sharing of information needs to be bilateral. You are expert on testing, treatment options and their outcomes and you need to convey this knowledge to the patient and family. The patient is the expert on their preferences and needs to convey this information to you.

Work **with** patients to establish doable goals to which they can wholeheartedly commit.

Here's how collaborative goal-setting might sound:

- **Doctor:** "So what are you thinking you can do this week to manage your reflux while you also begin taking the pills?"
- **Patient:** "I can eat right. I guess I'm eating the wrong things."
- **Doctor:** "That would be good. What exactly are you thinking about how you will eat differently?"
- **Patient:** "I'll just stop all sugar and fried foods, and I won't drink."
- **Doctor:** "All of those things WOULD help. I'm just wondering if those are too many changes to make at once?"
- **Patient:** "Well, I know if I cut out all of that, I would feel really sorry for myself and blow it."
- **Doctor:** "So, what might be a way to ease into this kind of eating in a way you can handle that won't make you feel sorry for yourself?"
- **Patient:** "Well I could start by getting rid of all sugar. I eat a load of it everyday and lots of chocolate."
- **Doctor:** "Being really realistic, what could you do to reduce your sugar and not feel like you're totally depriving yourself of what you like?"
- **Patient:** "I could stop drinking sodas and drink water instead. And I could limit myself to one candy bar a day. That's down from about three. And I could try to break my habit of ordering fried foods when I eat out. I don't care that much about them anyway and yet I eat them all the time."
- **Doctor:** "Sounds like a very good place to start. Let me write that down for you…. Drink water instead of sodas, one candy bar a day, and don't order fried foods when you eat out."
- **Patient:** "Yes!"
- **Doctor:** "Sounds good. You know Angie, my assistant?"
- **Patient:** "Yes."
- **Doctor:** "I'd like to ask Angie to call you at the end of next week to see how you're doing and she can let me know? I want to help you make your plan work, so you get that reflux under control."

While it might take more time to engage the patient in goal-setting, if you don't take that time, you risk being ineffective.

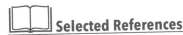 **Selected References**

1. Barry M, Shared decision-making: Informing and involving patients to do the right thing in health care. **J Ambulatory Care Management**; (2012) 35, 2, 90-98.

2. Berwick DM. What patient-centered should mean: Confessions of an extremist. **Health Aff**; (Millwood) 2009; 28: w555-w565.

3. Coleman MT, Newton KS. Supporting self-management in patients with chronic illness. **Am Fam Physician**; 2005; (72)8:1503-1510.

4. Coulter A, **Engaging Patients in Health Care**. 2011; NY: NY: McGraw-Hill Education.

5. Fowler FJ et al., Informing and involving patients to improve the quality of medical decisions. **Health Affairs**; 2011; 390, 699-706.

6. Frosch D. et al., Authoritarian physicians and patients' fear of being labeled 'difficult' among key obstacles to shared decision making. **Health Affairs**; 5 (2012):1030–1038.

7. Institute for Healthcare Improvement, **Delivering Great Care: Engaging Patients and Families as Partners**; 2006. Available at www.IHI.org. Accessed October 24, 2012.

8. Lewin SA et al., Interventions for providers to promote a patient-centered approach in clinical consultations. **Cochrane Database of Systematic Reviews**; 2001; issue 4.

9. Michaud MD et al., Ten strategies to build partnerships with patients. **Wisconsin Med J**; 2007; 106, 8:444-446.

10. Patients as partners: How to involve patients and families in their own care. **Joint Commission Resources**;2006.

Self-Improvement Tools: Engaging Patients and Families as Partners

- **Personal Spot Check**
- **Patient Feedback**
- **Family Feedback**
- **Peer/Colleague Feedback**

Personal Spot-Check:
On Engaging Patients and Families as Partners

With this patient, which best practices did I use?	YES ✓
1. Did I encourage the patient to speak freely about his or her concerns before I intervened?	
2. Did I negotiate the visit agenda with the patient, instead of setting it myself?	
3. Did I invite the patient's ideas and viewpoints before making suggestions?	
4. Did I jointly discuss the patient's values and their impact on care options and decisions?	
5. Did I make a concerted effort to engage the patient in decisions about their care?	
6. If there were family members present, did I invite and address their questions and concerns?	

What one thing did I do especially well to engage my patient (and their family)?

What one thing do I want to do differently to be even more collaborative and patient-centered in my approach?

Patient Feedback:
On Engaging Patients and Families as Partners

Dear Patient,
I want to provide you with great care and service. It's very important to me to engage you as a partner in our talks and in decisions about your care. Please think about today's visit and tell me which of these actions I did today to work together with you. I welcome your feedback.

	YES ✓
1. Did I encourage you to speak freely about your concerns before I started talking?	
2. Did I plan the visit agenda with you, instead of setting it myself?	
3. Did I invite your ideas and views before making suggestions?	
4. Did we discuss what's most important to you about your care?	
5. Did I engage you in decisions about your care?	
6. If you had family members present, did I involve them in our conversation in an effective way?	

Please suggest one thing I can do in the future to be more effective. _____
_____
_____

THANK YOU!

Family Feedback:
On Engaging Patients and Families as Partners

Dear Family Member,
I want to provide you and the patient with exceptional care
and service. It's very important to me to engage with my patients'
family members as partners since your involvement and support is
so important to my patients' health results. Please think about
today's visit and tell me which of these actions I did to engage
with you for the patient's sake. I welcome your feedback.

	YES ✓
1. Did I make you feel welcome?	
2. Did I invite your questions and concerns?	
3. Did I address your questions and concerns?	
4. Did I involve you in the discussion as much as you wanted?	
5. Did I encourage the patient to speak freely about concerns before I gave advice?	
6. In the visit, did we address the patient's most important concerns?	
7. Did I listen to you well when you had things to say?	
8. If it was appropriate, did I involve you in decisions about the patient's care?	
9. Do you feel you could call me if you have a concern about the patient later?	

Please suggest one thing I can do in the future to be more effective. _____

_____

_____

THANK YOU!

Dear Colleague,
I'm committed to patient and family-centered care and I'm working
on more effectively engaging my patients and their family members
as partners. Please observe me and give me your feedback on how well I
do on patient and family engagement and offer your suggestions.
I welcome this.

	YES ✓
1. Did I encourage the patient to speak freely about concerns before I intervened?	
2. Did I plan the visit agenda with the patient (and family members), instead of setting it myself?	
3. Did I invite the patient's (and family member's) ideas and views before making suggestions?	
4. Did I engage the patient in decisions about their care?	
5. Did I use partnership language like "we" and "together" to encourage working together?	
6. If there were family members present, did I invite and address their questions?	
7. If there were family members present, did I involve them appropriately in sharing information and making decisions?	
8. Did you think I behaved in a collaborative way?	

What are your suggestions? _____

_____

_____

THANK YOU!

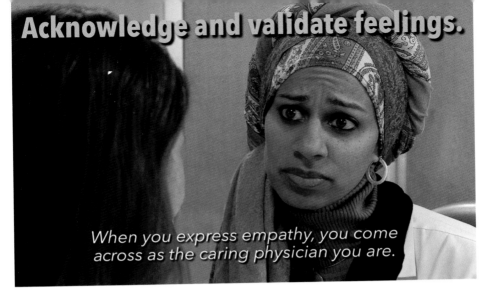

Acknowledge and validate feelings.

When you express empathy, you come across as the caring physician you are.

7. Communicating with Empathy

🔍 QUICK SELF-CHECK	YES ✓
1. Do I make sure I connect to the patient as a person?	
2. Do I watch for nonverbal clues about what the patient is feeling?	
3. Do I invite the patient to share his or her experience and feelings? ("I want to understand." "Did I miss anything?")	
4. Do I check out and acknowledge the patient's feelings using words like "you sound" or "you seem" (upset, concerned, relieved, confused, etc.), or "Let me see if I have this right"?	
5. Do I validate or confirm the legitimacy of the patients' feelings, showing my understanding?	
6. Do I express empathy to people different from myself as much as I do to people similar to me?	
7. Do I pursue or follow up on a patient's expressed feeling?	
8. If family members are present, do I connect with them personally?	
9. If family members are present, do I show empathy for their feelings too?	
10. Do I show empathy in my nonverbal behavior, by nodding, looking concerned, and the like?	

A physician competent and effective at displaying empathy replies YES to these questions. If you can't reply YES, note opportunities to improve the patient and family experience by mastering the skill of communicating with empathy.

When you communicate with empathy, patients benefit and so do you.

Working Definition of Empathy: Two Components

- **Understanding** the patient's experience, concerns and perspective
- **Acknowledging and validating** the patient's feelings

Empathy is often confused with 'sympathy." A sympathetic caregiver feels the feeling the patient is feeling. Their feelings are congruent. For example: The physician feels sad when the patient does, becomes teary when the patient cries, and feels vicarious anger when the patient tells of an injustice. While sympathy can contribute positively to the patient relationship, it can be exhausting. Also, some physicians might not feel sympathy if they experience the patient as unlikable, frustrating or 'different.'

The good news is that you can express empathy even without feeling sympathy and the positive effects are significant. The art of empathic presence doesn't involve emotional enmeshment.

Facts

- Physician empathy is strongly associated with patient satisfaction and trust.
- Empathic physicians score higher on HCAHPS and CG-CAHPS.
- The empathic physician is more likely to elicit the full story and this leads to more accurate diagnosis, treatment and support.
- Patients of empathic physicians show greater compliance and adherence and better outcomes for many acute and chronic conditions.
- Empathic physicians have higher job satisfaction, less stress and burnout, and far fewer lawsuits.

Patients want their physicians to be empathic.

- They feel understood, respected and valued.
- Their anxiety decreases.
- They become more engaged and are more likely to have positive outcomes.
- They are more positive about their experience.

Also, when you communicate empathy in patient encounters, you benefit.

- Because your relationship with your patients is more satisfying, so is your work.
- Your patient engages and achieves better outcomes.
- You receive high ratings from patients and this engenders professional pride as well as optimal earnings under pay-for-performance.

Empathy in medicine is scarce.

Did you know?

- Four out of 5 physicians ignore patients' clues and expressions of affect.
- Those who do respond shift quickly to biomedical issues.
- On top of that, while members of minority groups give empathic physicians much higher ratings than they give non-empathic physicians, physicians express far less empathy with patients from different cultures.

Signs That Empathy Is Lacking

Patients perceive a lack of empathy when you:

- Interrupt or finish the patient's thoughts
- Challenge the patient's feelings
- Reassure the patient in a way that sounds patronizing
- Tell the patient what they ought to think or feel
- Turn the topic to yourself and away from the patient

These behaviors shut the patient down and make them feel disregarded.

Based on the Evidence: Skills for Communicating with Empathy

Feeling empathy and expressing empathy are two different things. By following five rules of thumb, you can be sure that your inherent empathy will be felt by the people you serve.

You can communicate empathy with words, nonverbal behavior and, better yet, both together.

Five Rules of Thumb: Communicating with Empathy

1. Use the Heart-Head-Heart Sandwich Technique.

2. Acknowledge the person's feelings.

3. Follow up; pursue the patient or family member's feelings.

4. Validate or legitimize the patient or family member's feelings.

5. Show your empathy nonverbally.

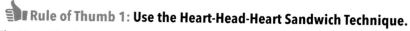 **Rule of Thumb 1: Use the Heart-Head-Heart Sandwich Technique.**

The Heart-Head-Heart Communication Model calls for two kinds of messages in your communication with patients and families. One message is a Heart message. It's personal and subjective -- about emotions and concerns. The other message is a Head message. It's about the task or problem at hand. It's more rational and information-oriented.

Two Kinds of Communication

Heart-to-Heart

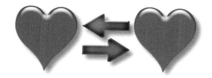

Emotion, Caring,
Empathy

Head-to-Head

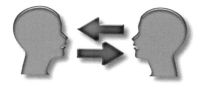

Tasks, Information,
Analysis, Questions,
Solutions

The fact is, both HEAD and HEART messages have benefits.

- When you express empathy—speaking from the heart, patients and families feel important. They feel your caring. Their anxiety decreases. And they can more easily absorb information.
- When you speak from your head--inquiring, analyzing and problem-solving--patients learn valuable information and they appreciate answers and solutions.

Here's the rub. These days, busy-ness and pressure make providers very task-oriented. Most communication is from the HEAD, much less from the HEART. If that's true of you, you can expect patients and families to view you as competent, but they might not feel your empathy and caring.

Consider a patient complaining loudly of pain. Many caregivers respond from the head—moving immediately to finding out more in an effort to fix the problem.

- How would you rate your pain?
- Where is the pain exactly?
- What seems to make it better or worse?
- I'll try you on some different medication.

These "head" responses help you identify the problem and move to remedies, but, without expressing empathy to the patient in response to their pain, the patient might very well experience you as unfeeling—helpful perhaps, but unfeeling.

The Ideal: The "Heart-Head-Heart Sandwich" Technique

- Start with HEART.
- Convey a HEAD message.
- End with HEART again.

Let's hear the Heart-Head-Heart Sandwich with our patient in pain:

Patient: "I'm having terrible pain!"

Physician:

- Heart: "I'm so sorry. I can see you're in terrible pain!"
- Head: "Tell me more about the pain."
- Heart: "I want to help."

Patients and families feel understood when you speak from the heart, showing regard for their feelings, not just for the content of what they say.

Consider this example:

Patient (exclaiming): "Haven't you done enough tests already!?"

Physician: "I just want three more tests."

The physician replied to the patient's words with a HEAD message and disregarded the patient's feelings.

Blending Heart with Head messages, this physician would be more effective if he or she were to respond with empathy, acknowledging and addressing the patient's feelings before addressing the facts, as follows:

"You sound really exhausted from this process. It's just that three more tests will be very helpful, and I want to get to the bottom of this for you."

Patients experience your expressions of empathy as HEART messages, and HEART messages on your part help patients and families feel your kindness, caring and support.

👍 Rule of Thumb 2: **Acknowledge the person's feelings.**

• Read the patient's (or family member's) words and nonverbal cues, and reflect back the feeling you think the person is feeling. • Sound tentative and curious, so the person can correct you if your reading of their feelings is not exactly right. • Be accepting, not judgmental.	• *"You sound worried?"* • *"You look unsure?"* • *"It sounds like this has been a tough decision for you."* • *"You look relieved!"*
Helpful Sentence Starters: • *"You sound.... "* • *"You seem.... "* • *"I imagine you might feel.... "*	**NO!:** • *"You shouldn't feel that way!"* • *"Now, don't jump to conclusions!"* • *"Whoa, you're getting ahead of yourself!"* **YES!:** • *"I'm so sorry it's upsetting."* • *"I realize it's scary."*

👍 Rule of Thumb 3: **Follow up. Pursue the patient or family member's feelings.**

Restate the feeling, checking with the patient or family member that you've understood.	**Physician:** *"Sounds like you're pretty frustrated with those exercises?* **Patient:** *"Yes, there are just too many!"* **Physician:** *"Let's take a look together and see how we can make them more doable for you."*
Ask the patient or family member a related question.	• *"What in particular is worrying you?"* • *"Tell me what's confusing, so I can help."*
Elaborate on a point the person made.	• *"There ARE a lot of ways we can approach this and each option has its pros and cons."*
Try to provide some comfort or relief from the feeling.	• *"Let's talk about what might ease your mind."* • *"How about if I make a list for you to make the steps much easier to follow?"*

👍 Rule of Thumb 4: **Validate or legitimize the patient or family member's feelings.**

Make a statement legitimizing the patient's emotion.	• *"You certainly have reason to feel exhausted."* • *"This IS a very hard decision to make."* • *"I can certainly understand that this is disturbing news."* • *"You have every reason to feel relieved!"*
Suggest that the person is not alone—that others have experienced this same feeling, progress or challenge.	• *"Others facing this feel a lot like you do."* • *"You're not alone in feeling this way."*
Listen intently, nodding with approval.	• *"I hear you."*
Make an affirming remark.	• *"This must be so difficult and you're very brave!"* • *"I realize your father's care requires a lot from you, and I think you're doing a really great job!"*

👍 Rule of Thumb 5: **Show Your Empathy Nonverbally.**

The fact is, you are never saying nothing, even when you're not talking. As shown in the following graphic, when your words and nonverbal behavior are out of sync, people believe your nonverbal behavior more than they believe your words.

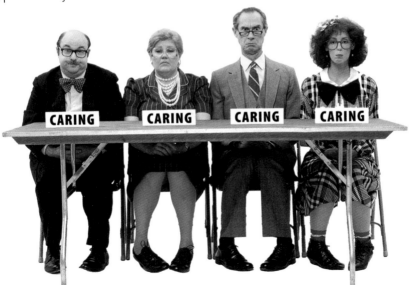

It is critical to make sure that your nonverbal behavior communicates empathy and caring.

- Extensive research points to one rule of thumb for showing empathy nonverbally. Take your cues from the other person and mirror their nonverbal behaviors.

- When you match your nonverbal behaviors to those of the other person, you appear empathic. In the literature on nonverbal behavior, this is called **"nonverbal listening," "attunement,"** or **"nonverbal reciprocity."**

Examples	
Looking angry, a patient exclaims: *"When she took my blood, she tore up my arm!"*	The physician matches the patient's look of anger with a very similar look of intense concern.
You're running late. The patient has been waiting, wondering and perhaps stewing about when you'll arrive.	Knowing that the patient is likely to be feeling a sense of urgency (or worse), enter the room showing urgency on your face and enter with a quickened pace.

And be sure to show empathy with people from other cultures.

Take your cues from them. Their behavior will show you what is comfortable for them. If you sustain eye contact and they look away, look away. If they step back a bit, step back a bit. And when in doubt, show respect and ask what makes them comfortable.

Physician: "I want to be sure I'm respectful of any cultural concerns or information that might affect you or your care. I don't know your culture very well. Please help me. I need you to tell me…."

View communicating with empathy as a feedback loop.

Empathic communication requires a series of back-and-forth communications that help the patient get clear and that help you verify your understanding.

The Feedback Loop in Action:

1. The patient speaks.
2. You listen with sustained eye contact, mirroring the person's facial expression and silence mixed "Hmmm" and "Uh-huh".
3. You encourage more talking ("Tell me more." Or, "I can only imagine how hard it is for you.")
4. You check out your understanding. "Let me see if I have this right." "Sounds like …"
5. You reflect back the content part of the patient's message. "So, you felt well until last night and during the night your pain got worse and kept you up."
6. And if the patient doesn't express feelings, but you know they must be having them, then invite the patient to express their feelings. "Tell me how you're feeling about all of this." Or, "I imagine this could raise some strong feelings for you. What ARE you feeling?"

7. Then, respond to the feelings you're hearing.
   - **To sadness:** "That sounds really painful and you sound very sad about it."
   - **Distrust:** "You seem concerned about whether you can rely on me since you had so much trouble reaching me."
   - **Mixed feelings:** "You sound pulled between wanting to lose weight and feeling hopeless about it."
   - **Anger:** "That experience sounds like it really made you angry, and I can certainly understand that."
8. And finally, ask for and accept corrections. "I want to understand. Did I miss anything?"

The process goes on until you hear a reassuring "That's it. You got it!"

Wrap-Up

Even though you care deeply, patients and families and your colleagues don't know it unless you communicate your empathy---both verbally and nonverbally. By using the skills described here, you can be sure they will feel your caring.

Rules of Thumb: Communicating with Empathy

1. Use the Heart-Head-Heart Sandwich Technique	• **HEART first:** Communicate with empathy. Address the person's feelings and anxieties. • **Then HEAD:** Address the issue or task at hand. Convey information. • **HEART last:** Close on a personal or feeling note.
2. Acknowledge the person's feelings.	• Read the patient's (or their family member's) words and nonverbal cues and reflect back the feeling you think you are seeing or hearing. • Sound tentative, so the person can clarify. • Be accepting and nonjudgmental.
3. Pursue: **Follow up on the feeling.**	• Ask the patient or family member a related question. • Elaborate on a point made. • Try to provide some comfort or relief from uncomfortable feelings.
4. Validate: **Legitimize the feeling.**	• Acknowledge that a challenge is difficult. • Suggest that others have had a similar experience. • Listen intently, nodding with approval. • Make a congratulatory or appreciative remark.
5. Show empathy nonverbally.	Mirror: Match your nonverbal behavior to that of the other person. • Meet anger with a look of concern. • Meet urgency with urgency. • Meet calm with calm. Adjust your eyes, posture, pace and face to mirror the other person.

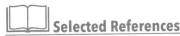 **Selected References**

1. Back A et al., **Mastering Communication with Seriously Ill Patients: Balancing Honesty with Empathy and Hope**. New York: Cambridge Univ Pr;2009.

2. Churchill LR and Schenck D, Healing skills for medical practice. **Ann Intern Med**; 2008;149:720-4.

3. Coulehan JL et al., Let me see if I have this right: Words that help build empathy. **Ann Intern Med**; August 7, 2001;135:221-227

4. Easter DW, Beach W, Competent patient care is dependent upon attending to empathic opportunities presented during interview sessions. **Curr Surg**; 2004;61:313-8.

5. Fadiman A, **The Spirit Catches You and You Fall Down: A Hmong Child, Her American Doctors, and the Collision of Two Cultures**. NY: Farrar, Straus and Giroux;1997.

6. Fogarty LA et al., Can 40 seconds of compassion reduce patient anxiety? **J Clin Oncol;**17:371-379.

7. Frenkel DN and Liebman CB, Words that heal. **Ann Int Med**;140(6): 482-483.

8. Halpern J, Empathy and patient-physician conflicts. **J Gen Intern Med**; 2007;22:696-700.

9. Schattner A, Who cares for empathy? **QJM**; 2012;105(3):287-290.

10. Schattner A, The silent dimension. Expressing humanism in each medical encounter. **Arch Intern Med**;2009;169:1095-9.

Self-Improvement Tools: Communicating with Empathy

- **Personal Spot Check**
- **Patient Feedback**
- **Family Feedback**
- **Peer/Colleague Feedback**

With this patient, which best practices did I use?	YES ✓
1. I made sure I connected to the patient as a person.	
2. I invited the patient to share his or her experience and feelings.	
3. I acknowledged the patient's feelings using words like, "you sound" or "you seem…" (upset, concerned, relieved, confused).	
4. I validated or confirmed the legitimacy of the patient's feelings.	
5. I followed up on the patient's feelings.	
6. If family members were present, I showed understanding of their feelings.	
7. I showed empathy in my nonverbal behavior (e.g. by nodding, looking concerned, or scrunching my forehead).	

What did I do well?

What do I want to do differently to be even more effective in showing empathy?

Dear Patient,
I want to provide you with excellent medical care in a personal and
compassionate manner. Will you please think about our conversation
today and give me feedback. I welcome it.

	YES ✓
1. Did I connect with you personally?	
2. Did I invite you to talk about your experience and feelings?	
3. Did I acknowledge or show understanding of your feelings?	
4. Did I accept your feelings, without judging?	
5. Did I address your feelings or follow up on them?	
6. If family members were present, did I connect with them personally?	
7. If family members were present, did I show understanding of their feelings?	

Overall, how was my empathy today? _____

_____

_____

Please suggest one thing I can do in the future to be more effective? _____

_____

_____

THANK YOU!

Dear Family Member,
I want to provide you and the patients with exceptional care and service.
Right now, I'm working on communicating with empathy in conversations
with patients and families. Will you please think about our conversation
today and give me feedback. I welcome it.

	YES ✓
1. Did I connect with the patient personally?	
2. Did I invite the patient to talk about his or her experience and feelings?	
3. Did I acknowledge the patient's feelings?	
4. Did I show acceptance of the patient's feelings, without judging?	
5. Did I follow up on the patient's feelings?	
6. Did I show empathy for YOUR feelings?	
7. Overall, how well did I show empathy?	

Please suggest one thing I can do in the future to be more effective. _____
_____
_____

THANK YOU!

Dear Colleague,
I want to provide our patients and families with exceptional care.
Right now, I'm working on communicating with empathy. You were
present with me during an encounter today. Will you please reflect on
your observations? I'll appreciate your feedback.

	YES ✓
1. Did I connect with the patient/family personally?	
2. Did I invite the patient/family to talk about their experience and feelings?	
3. Did I acknowledge the patient's feelings?	
4. Did I show acceptance of people's feelings, without judging?	
5. Overall, how well did I show empathy?	
6. If family members were present, did I connect with them personally?	
7. If family members were present, did I show understanding of their feelings?	
8. In my interactions with YOU, did I treat YOU with empathy and respect?	

What are your suggestions? _____

_____

_____

THANK YOU!

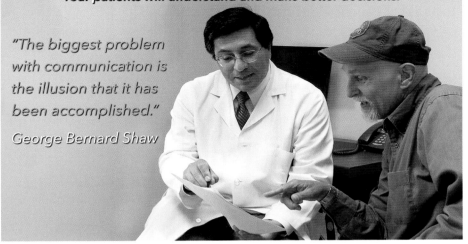

Ask-Tell-Ask.
Your patients will understand and make better decisions.

"The biggest problem with communication is the illusion that it has been accomplished."

George Bernard Shaw

8. Effective Explanations

🔍 QUICK SELF-CHECK	YES ✓
1. Do I ask the patient how much they want to know and honor their preference?	
2. Do I find out from the patient what they already know, so I can build on this and address misinformation?	
3. Do I avoid using acronyms and jargon, so patients can more easily understand me?	
4. Do I encourage questions as I proceed with an explanation?	
5. Do I find out what people have understood, instead of taking for granted that they've understood me?	
6. Do I use the "Teach Back" technique to find out what patients and their family members have heard and understood?	
7. When family members are present, do I make sure they leave understanding how they can help?	

Physicians who are competent, thorough, respectful and effective at explaining respond YES to all eight statements.

Facts about Patient Absorption of Information

- Patients and families have overwhelming access to information---from the internet, direct-to-consumer advertising, friends and family, talk shows and the like, and they come to you much more informed (and sometimes misinformed) than ever.
- Patients understand less than half of what their physicians explain to them.
- In a study by Castro (2007), 81% of encounters contained at least one unclarified jargon term (a mean of 4 per visit). Thirty-seven percent of jargon use occurred when making recommendations and 29% when providing health education. Patient comprehension rates were generally low and never reached adequate thresholds.
- Many patients leave medical encounters with a poor understanding of their disease and the recommended treatment.
- Hewson (1993) found that, when patients were asked to explain what they'd heard from their doctor, their explanations included many gaps and errors indicating retention of less than half of the information.
- Britten's study (2000) of twenty general practices revealed that, in 80% of the encounters, misunderstandings occurred that related to actual or potential adverse outcomes.

Note that CAHPS surveys ask your patients about the effectiveness of your explanations.

- The HCAHPS survey asks: "During this hospital stay, how often did the doctor EXPLAIN THINGS in a way you could understand?"
- The CG-CAHPS Survey includes:
    › "Providers explained things in a way that was easy to understand."
    › "Providers gave easy to understand information about health questions or concerns."

The High Cost of Ineffective Explanations

When medical explanations are inaccurate, unclear, incomplete or overwhelming, patients and families, the society and physicians pay a high price.

"Physicians who fail to verify patient understanding of medical information run a greater risk of negative patient outcomes as well as malpractice claims. And, the society as a whole absorbs an estimated $73 billion annually because of misunderstood medical information." (Kemp et al., 2008)

Your effectiveness at explaining impacts your effectiveness in securing:

* Informed consent
* Patient safety
* Patient and family comprehension of options and follow-up care
* Patient commitment and adherence
* Positive outcomes
* Patient satisfaction with you and the clinical encounter

Effective Explanations: Simple, But Not Easy

Even when your knowledge is impeccable, it's not easy to explain effectively.

- Many patients are anxious, fearful or intimidated. This makes it hard for them to listen and absorb what you're saying.
- People come to you with preconceived notions and they might filter what you're saying through these preconceived ideas or leanings.
- Differences in cultural background, education level, language, hearing, health literacy, family health history, and how much each person wants to know, affect people's comprehension, making it critical to tailor explanations to the individual.

Behaviors to Avoid	Examples
Talking too fast	"With blood pressure medication, there can be side effects. If you're taking too much, it could drive your blood pressure down too much. It might make you dizzy. It could make you feel tired. It could slow your heartbeat. You might not be able to perform sexually, but it shouldn't interfere with the other meds you're taking."
Jargon and acronyms	• "Your EKG shows an elongated QT interval, so we'll do an ECHO and serial EKGs." • "You'll go to the OR and from there to the PACU and from there to either Med-Surg or the ICU." • "You can have your pain medicine PRN." • "Are you having pain in your right upper quadrant?" • "Your test results are positive" (which might be good or bad). • "The mass is benign." • "CABG due to myocardial infarction."
Talking down to the patient	**Patient:** "My sister got diabetes when she was pregnant. Will I get it too?" **Physician:** (patting the patient's shoulder): "I don't want you to worry about things like that. Just go home and have a nice baby, and I'll take care of this."
Talking louder in the face of a language barrier	**Patient:** "No comprendo." **Physician:** Repeats the same point again in the same words, but much more loudly
Interrupting and discouraging questions	**Patient:** starting to ask a question **Physician:** (on the way to the door) "There's a bowel prep you need to do. The instructions are in the box. Get here an hour early and I'll see you in the OR."
Explaining too much at a time	Rule of thumb: No more than three bits of information at once.

Based on the Evidence: ASK-TELL-ASK

Substantial research over the last thirty years has established an evidence base for the ASK-TELL-ASK approach as the state-of-the-art approach to explaining effectively.

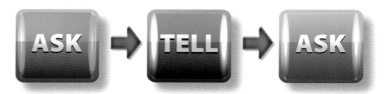

- ASK: Find out what the person already knows and wants to know.
- TELL: Provide your explanation to meet the person's information needs.
- ASK: Verify understanding and address information gaps, questions and concerns.

The First Step: ASK

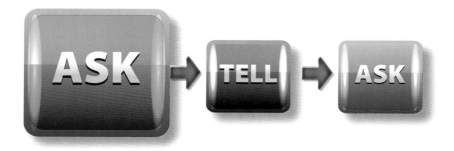

Ask before telling. Start with questions, not information. Listen carefully. This will help you tailor your explanation to the individual's knowledge, questions and concerns.

Rules of Thumb	**Examples**
1. Encourage the patient (and family) to ask questions at any time during your explanation.	• *"I want to do a good job explaining this, so please tell me when I say anything that isn't clear to you."* • *"Please speak up if I'm not clear. That would really help me."*
2. Then, elicit the patient's knowledge. *Get grounded in what the patient already knows so you build on their knowledge and also correct what might be misinformation.*	**Doctor:** *"So, this is the first time you're hearing about your diabetes. Do you know anyone who has diabetes?"* **Patient:** *"My aunt has it."* **Doctor:** *"Tell me, what's your understanding of it?"* **Doctor:** *"Have you done any reading about this, like on the internet? If so, what struck you as important?"*
3. Invite the patient (and family) to express their concerns. *Probe for these so you can tailor your explanation to address not only key information but also the patient's (and family's) anxieties and concerns.*	*"How are you feeling about this?"* *"What's concerning you the most?"* **Patient:** *"My aunt has diabetes and she has to watch her sugars and be careful about her food. And she worries about her kidneys. I think it's made her really sick."* **Doctor:** *"How worried are you that this might affect you the way it's affected your aunt?"* **Patient:** *"Very worried."* **Doctor:** *"What else is worrying you?"*

The Second Step: TELL

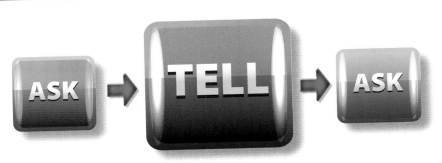

After you lay the groundwork by asking questions, then comes the explanation itself…. The TELL step.

🖐 Rules of Thumb	Examples
1. If there's a language barrier, bring in a *trained* translator. *Don't rely on family members because you can't be sure if their translations will reflect what you're saying or their own preconceived ideas or concerns.*	A loving wife might not want to tell her husband what the physician actually said, because she thinks it will upset him.
2. As you begin to explain, state your purpose or positive intent. *Make it personal---all about the patient!*	• *"I'm ordering this blood work to see if we can find a reason for your tiredness."* • *"Ms. Parks? This is Dr. Turner. I'm calling to ease your mind about your test results!"* • *"I want to talk with you about your alcohol use, because I want to help you live a long, healthy life."* • *"I want to get to the bottom of this with you."*
3. Explain in a way that is easy to understand. *Medical explanations can be as clear as mud. Avoid jargon and acronyms.*	<table><tr><th>Jargon</th><th>Plain Talk</th></tr><tr><td>Modify</td><td>*Change*</td></tr><tr><td>Benign</td><td>*Not cancer*</td></tr><tr><td>Fracture</td><td>*Break*</td></tr><tr><td>Hypertension</td><td>*High blood pressure*</td></tr><tr><td>Interaction</td><td>*How things work together*</td></tr><tr><td>Intermittent</td><td>*Off and on*</td></tr><tr><td>Lesion</td><td>*Wound; sore*</td></tr><tr><td>Enlarge</td><td>*Get bigger*</td></tr><tr><td>Oral</td><td>*By mouth*</td></tr><tr><td>Optimal</td><td>*Best*</td></tr></table>

👍 **Rules of Thumb**	**Examples**
4. Use metaphors and analogies to foster clarity and retention. *"Metaphors may be as necessary to illness as they are to literature, as comforting to the patient as his own bathrobe and slippers. At the very least, they are a relief from medical terminology. Perhaps only metaphor can express the bafflement, the panic combined with beatitude, of the threatened person."* *Anatole Broyard*	Make the strange familiar. • *Immune system as "the defending army"* • *"The rash is like a sunburn."* • *"After a bone marrow transplant, you will feel like you were kicked by a horse."* • *"It's like drinking a milkshake."* • *"It's the size of a pea."* • *"The therapy is more like a marathon than a sprint."* • *"I see two options for you. One puts you in low gear and the other in high gear."* Also, use drawings along with your words–e.g. drawings from the world of machines, plumbing, sports and the like.
5. Be sure to address the **"what ifs."** Patients wonder, *"What if this happens?"* If you don't address the **what ifs**, these concerns make patients and family members anxious later and much more likely to call you for support or more information.	**Physician:** *"If your symptoms return, here's what to do…"* **Physician:** *"If you find yourself too sleepy during the day, then please call me and we'll try something else."* **Physician:** *"If we don't get the answer from the test, here's what we'll do next to figure out what's going on."*
6. Go beyond facts. Address the patient's (and family's) questions and anxieties with empathy and caring.	**Physician:** *"I realize this might sound frightening."* **Physician:** *"And you said you were concerned about whether you could work during your recovery. I realize --6 weeks IS a long time to be off work."*
7. Don't overwhelm. • Give no more than 3 bits of information at once, before checking understanding. • Watch for signs of inattention, confusion or overload. Check in before going on.	*"You look a little puzzled?"* or *"What are you thinking?"* **Physician:** *"I'm going to have you do a 24-hour urine collection for protein."* **Patient:** *Responds with furrowed eyebrows and a look of dismay.* **Physician:** *"You look unsure. Let me explain what I mean and how this works."*

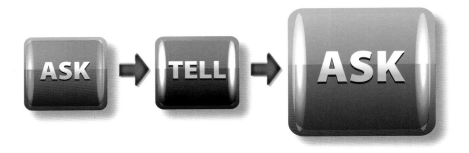

During the last step–the ASK step, find out what the patient has understood. This is critical to quality care and outcomes.

If you complete your explanation and the patient hasn't understood you, you have not been effective. And you can expect negative results---patient anxiety and lack of adherence, medication errors, missed appointments, adverse medical outcomes, and lawsuits.

EC. Kemp et al. (2008) researched the three most common ways physicians check patient understanding.

1. Yes-no	*"I've given you a lot of information. Do you understand?"*
2. Tell back-collaborative	*"I imagine you're really worried about this clot. I've given you a lot of information. It would be helpful to me to hear your understanding about your clot and its treatment."*
3. Tell back-directive	*"It's really important that you do this exactly the way I explained. What do you understand?"*

Kemp et al. found unequivocally that patients prefer **#2 -- the "Tell Back-Collaborative" method**. This method engages patients and produces the most positive patient outcomes.

👍 **Rules of Thumb**	**Examples**
1. To determine understanding, ask open-ended, not short-answer questions. *Closed-ended or "yes-no" questions tell you nothing about what the patient understands or doesn't.* • *If you ask, "Is that clear?" or "Do you understand?", most people will say "yes" even if it isn't clear, because they don't want to appear slow. Others will say "yes" because they think they understand, but they really don't.*	• *"What questions do you have? I want to hear."* • *"What can I go over so you feel really clear about what's going on?"* • *"What problems do you foresee with this plan?"*
2. Use the "Teach-Back" technique (sometimes called the Tell-Back Collaborative Method). *Ask the person to restate what you've told them in their own words. As you ask, sound supportive and nonthreatening, so the patient doesn't feel tested or embarrassed.*	• *"I want to be sure I've explained this well. At this point, what's your understanding of your condition?"* • *"I want to be sure I've been clear. What do you understand to be the most important things to do when you get home?"* • *"Okay, Mr. Simpson, I bet when you get home, your daughter will ask you what we talked about today. What are you going to tell her?"*
3. Listen; clarify any information gaps or misunderstandings, and check understanding again. *Just because you re-explain, it doesn't mean the person will comprehend this time. After listening carefully to their teach-back, tactfully re-explain or augment their understanding as needed.*	• *"Yes, and I just want to emphasize one important thing that I might not have explained well enough…"*

Beyond Your Communication Skills:
Provide Supplemental Communication Aids

You have limited time and cannot personally provide endless information and answers. Also, people learn and retain information in different ways, some visually and some verbally. That's why providing additional communication aids is so important. For the most common conditions you treat, be prepared to offer patients and families printed materials, visual aids, checklists, a list of quality YouTube videos and websites (WEBMD, MAYO, et al.) where they can expand their knowledge and reinforce the information you can provide personally. You can also subscribe to one of the myriad information services available to physicians for their patients.

Wrap-Up

Consider again George Bernard Shaw's wise words: *"The biggest problem with communication is the illusion that it has been accomplished."*

By using the **ASK-TELL-ASK** process, you can make sure you've been understood and help the patient and family achieve the best possible outcomes.

Highlights for Review

Effective Explanations with Patients and Families

ASK
- How much do you want to know?
- What do you already know?
- Please tell me your questions and concerns.

TELL
- State your positive intent.
- Make it easy to understand.
- Adress the "what ifs".
- Go beyond facts: Address anxieties.
- Watch for signs of confusion or overload.

ASK
- Check comprehension with open-ended, not short-answer questions.
- Use the "Teach-Back" technique.
- Listen; address information gaps and misunderstandings; check again.

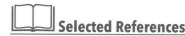 **Selected References**

1. Britten N et al., Misunderstandings in prescribing decisions in general practice: Qualitative study. **BMJ**;2000;320:484–8.
2. Casarett D et al., Can metaphors and analogies improve communication with seriously ill patients? **J Palliative Med**;13(3);2010.
3. Castro CM et al., Babel babble: Physicians' use of unclarified medical jargon with patients. **Am J Health Behav**;2007;31(Suppl 1):S85–S95.
4. Hewson MG, Patient education through teaching for conceptual change. **J Gen Intern Med**;1993;8:393–8.
5. Kemp EC et al., Patients prefer the method of "Tell Back- Collaborative Inquiry" to assess understanding of medical information. **J Am Board Fam Med**;2008;21(1):24-30.
6. Kripalani, S et al., Health literacy and the quality of physician-patient communication during hospitalization. **J Hospital Medicine**;5 (5);2010.
7. Periyakoil V, Using metaphors in medicine. **J Palliative Med**;11(6);2008.
8. Pfizer, The Newest Vital Sign: Health Literacy. Clear Health Communication Initiative; www.pfizerhealthliteracy.com. Accessed October 24, 2012.

Self-Improvement Tools: On Effective Explanations

- **Personal Spot Check**
- **Patient Feedback**
- **Family Feedback**
- **Peer/Colleague Feedback**

With this patient, which best practices did I use?	YES ✓
1. Did I ask the patient how much he or she wanted to know and honor this preference?	
2. Did I find out from the patient what he or she already knew, so I could build on this and address misinformation?	
3. Did I avoid using acronyms and jargon, so this patient could easily understand me?	
4. Did I make a point of encouraging questions?	
5. Did I speak respectfully to the patient and not talk down to them?	
6. Did I check out the patient's understanding using the Teach-Back technique?	
7. If family members were present, did I make sure I addressed their information needs effectively as well?	

What one thing did I do well?

What one thing do I want to do differently to be more effective with my explanations?

Patient Feedback: On Effective Explanations

Dear Patient,
I want to provide you with great care and service. It's very important to
me to explain things to you well, so that you feel clear. Will you please
think about how I explained things to you today and give me feedback. I
welcome it.

	YES ✓
1. Did I give you the information you wanted?	
2. Did I find out what you already knew before I explained things to you, so I could build on that?	
3. Did I explain things clearly so that I was easy to understand?	
4. Did I encourage you to ask questions?	
5. Did I check to make sure you felt clear about what we discussed?	
6. Did I explain everything you needed to know to feel prepared for your next steps?	

Please suggest one thing I can do in the future to be more effective when I explain things. _____
_____
_____

THANK YOU!

Family Feedback: On Effective Explanations

Dear Family Member,
I want to provide you and the patients with exceptional care and service.
Right now, I'm working on improving how I explain things to patients and
families. I want to provide effective explanations, so you and the patient
feel clear and respected and also prepared for your next steps. Please think
about how I explained things today and give me feedback. I welcome it.

	YES ✓
1. Did I give you and the patient the information you wanted?	
2. Did I find out what the patient already knew before I explained things?	
3. Did I explain things clearly, not using unfamiliar terms?	
4. Did I make a point of encouraging the patient to ask questions?	
5. Did I make a point of encouraging YOU to ask questions?	
6. Did I address YOUR information needs well?	
7. Did I check to make sure you and the patient felt clear about what we discussed?	

Please suggest one thing I can do in the future to be more effective when I provide explanations.

_____

_____

THANK YOU!

Dear Colleague,
I'm working on improving how I explain things to patients and families.
I want to provide effective explanations, so my patients and families feel
clear and respected and also prepared for their next steps. Please observe
my explanations during this visit and give me your feedback. I welcome it.

	YES ✓
1. Did I ask the patient how much he or she wanted to know and honor this preference?	
2. Did I find out what the patient already knew, so I could build on this and address misinformation?	
3. Did I avoid using acronyms and jargon, so the patient could easily understand me?	
4. Did I make a point of encouraging the patient to ask questions?	
5. Did I check for understanding, instead of taking for granted that the patient understood me?	
6. Did I use the "Teach Back" technique to check the patient's understanding?	
7. If family members were present, did I address their information needs as well?	
8. Did you think I behaved in a collaborative way?	

What are your suggestions? _____

_____

_____

THANK YOU!

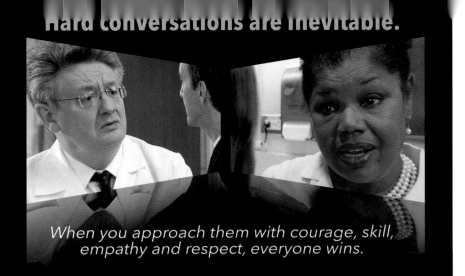

Hard conversations are inevitable.

When you approach them with courage, skill, empathy and respect, everyone wins.

9. Hard Conversations

QUICK SELF-CHECK	YES ✓
1. When I have an issue with a colleague's actions, do I address it directly with that person?	
2. When I have bad news to share with a patient, do I plan my approach so I'm more likely to handle it well?	
3. When I'm about to initiate a hard conversation, do I adjust my mindset, so I can approach the person in a positive, or at least a neutral frame of mind?	
4. Do I start a hard conversation with a positive statement of my hope or purpose for the conversation?	
5. Do I make my point quickly, instead of beating around the bush?	
6. Do I listen with an open mind to the other person's point of view?	
7. Do I try to achieve common ground with the other person, so we can agree on a plan moving forward?	
8. If the other person is resistant, do I remain caring in my manner?	
9. Do I express my appreciation to the other person for hearing me out?	
10. When someone initiates a hard conversation with me, do I listen with an open mind instead of becoming defensive?	

Skillful handling of hard conversations requires all of the above elements. Questions you answered with a NO provide clues to ways you can make your hard conversations consistently straightforward, respectful, and effective.

Facing the Inevitable: Hard Conversations

As you well know, hard conversations are inevitable in medicine.

- Telling a patient something they don't want to hear
- Confronting a coworker who's letting you or a patient down
- Saying "no" to a family member's request
- Handling a complaint
- Breaking bad news to a patient and their family
- Raising a touchy issue with a patient/family
- Giving an unwelcome instruction or suggestion
- Saying "no" to a colleague's unreasonable expectation

Presented with the need for a hard conversation, it's not unusual for physicians to bristle.

- "I'm fine with hard conversations with my patients, but when people I work with don't do what they promise, I have no patience for it."
- "I hate conflict. I just want to run the other way."
- "Patients come to me worried about their health. But when I tell them what they need to do, they don't listen."

Hard conversations, while inevitable, can be very stressful to anticipate and to carry out. And many people go to great lengths to avoid such conversations.

What stops us from entering into hard conversations when we have concerns that need addressing?

- We want to protect ourselves from embarrassment
- We might not have had much success handling hard conversations in the past
- We want to be nice, so we make allowances
- We procrastinate--because of anxiety
- We worry, "What if I don't handle it well and it makes matters worse?"

The fact is, if you avoid hard conversations when they're called for, this can preoccupy you and drain your energy. And nothing changes either. Patients and families miss out on your knowledge and perspective. And with coworkers, you pay a steep price...and so do your patients and your practice.

On the other hand, when you handle hard conversations well, everyone benefits.

- Patients and families feel respected by you and respect you for your forthright approach. They're more likely to engage and commit to their care plan. And this results in better outcomes.
- Colleagues respect you and are more likely to cooperate and support you, and
- You benefit -- by earning respect, by enjoying harmonious relationships, and by achieving better results. Also, you reduce the stress and distress in your inherently stressful job.

This section presents a straightforward, evidence-based approach to handling hard conversations, so that they are constructive and respectful, easier to initiate and endure, and most likely to achieve the results you want. We want to refresh the skills that make hard conversations easier. We're not going to address breaking bad news, because that's a whole topic unto itself, but we will address skills that can help you break bad news and also handle many other challenging situations with patients and coworkers.

 ## The Best Practice Approach to Hard Conversations

The Goal: Handle hard conversations in a manner that is constructive and respectful, easy to initiate and endure, and most likely to achieve the results you want.

👍 Four Rules of Thumb: Hard Conversations

1. Adopt a helpful mindset.

2. Follow the Hard Conversations Model.

3. Address resistance with the Caring Broken Record.

4. When you're on the receiving end, open your mind.

👍 Rule of Thumb 1: **Adopt a helpful mindset.**

Before jumping into a hard conversation, make sure you enter the conversation in a positive or at least a neutral frame of mind. If you feel apprehension, anger or blame, this makes it very hard to approach a person in a constructive and caring way.

Imagine approaching a hard conversation with thoughts like these:

- "I've had it with this person."
- "Here they go again."
- "Don't blame me!"
- "I can't wait to get THIS over with."
- "They are going to be furious about this!"
- "What an impossible person!"
- "They have no respect for me."
- "I have no respect for them."

Thoughts like these will make it very hard to approach the other person in a calm, caring and constructive manner.

As hard as it may be, you need to find a way to adopt an attitude of appreciation and goodwill.

- If you feel apprehension, anger or blame, shake it off.
- Adopt an attitude of respect, openness and inquiry.
- In your mind, give the other person the benefit of the doubt. Assume they mean well and mean you no harm.
- Put yourself in the other person's place.

Talk to yourself. Tell yourself constructive thoughts like these:

- "He means well."
- "For all I know, he could be clueless."
- "No risk, no gain."
- "The past is the past. Maybe the time is now."
- "He probably does care about his relationship with me."
- "She wants to do the right thing."

👍 Rule of Thumb 2: Follow the Hard Conversations Model.

Use the six-step *Hard Conversations Model* to plan and conduct an effective conversation.

The Hard Conversations Model

Step ❶: Upfront, state your positive intent first.
Step ❷: Tell the truth fast.
Step ❸: Listen and understand.
Step ❹: Find common ground.
Step ❺: Identify options and your action plan.
Step ❻: Express appreciation.

More about Each Step

Step	Tips	Sample Words
Step ❶: **Upfront, state your positive intent first.** *Don't begin by complimenting the other person, being extra-nice, or reassuring. People experience these openings as sugar-coated spitballs; they brace themselves for what's coming, and you minimize the importance of your message.*	• Explain what you're hoping to achieve in the conversation. • Do so in a direct and positive way.	• Physician to nurse: "I want to work with you to take the best possible care of our patients." • Physician to patient: "I want to help you solve the problem with your cough, so you can lead a long, healthy life." • Physician to colleague: "I want a good, collaborative relationship with you."

Step	Tips	Sample Words
Step ❷: **Tell the truth fast.**	• Spill the beans right away-- the facts, events or circumstances. Be factual and specific. Don't beat around the bush. • Explain why it's a problem--its consequences and results	• Physician to patient: "I'm worried about your weight. It's causing pressure on your knees and adding to your pain." • Physician to colleague: "You seem distracted. I'm concerned about how you're interacting with patients."
Step ❸: **Listen and understand.**	• Invite the person's reactions. Open your mind. And as you listen, consider the possibility that you might be wrong.	• Physician to patient: "Tell me how you see it. I want to understand." • Physician to colleague: "Perhaps you see it differently? Tell me."
	• Acknowledge the person's feelings and empathize.	• Physician to patient: "I realize your weight has plagued you and you've tried diets many times." • Physician to colleague: "I recognize that you have a lot going on in your life that makes it hard to focus."
	• Probe and ask clarifying questions.	• Physician to patient: "How do you feel about this?" • Physician to patient: "Tell me more about what made that hard?"
	• Check your understanding, so you're on the same page before you proceed.	• Physician to patient: "So, you're saying you've tried many times and feel hopeless?" • Physician to patient: "Let me see if I got that right?"
Step ❹: **Find common ground.**	• Finding common ground is so important. This conversation should not feel like a "you against me" experience. If you have a shared goal, you'll be better able to generate solutions that will work for BOTH of you.	• "We both want the same thing. We want you to be as happy and healthy as you can be...." • "We both want what's best for patients."

Step	Tips	Sample Words
Step ⑤: **Identify options and your action plan.**	• Generate several ideas together before settling on any one. What can YOU do? What can the other person do? What can you do together? • Discuss the pros and cons of each option and work toward a plan in a respectful give-and-take fashion.	• Physician: "So, after talking with you about how to proceed, here's what we agreed to…" • Patient: "So, what I think will work the best is for me to meet with the health coach you're recommending and work out a concrete plan."
Step ⑥: **Express appreciation.**	• Express your regard for the other person, because, despite being nervous, this person listened to you and worked with you to find a better way.	• "I know you care about our patients and I appreciate your understanding." • "Thank you for working with me on this. I realize it wasn't easy to hear."

Example: A primary care physician initiates a hard conversation, first adjusting his mindset to a positive one and then using the 6-Step Hard Conversations Model.

The Situation: A parent calls her son's physician and asks him to complete Jimmy's camp form and fax it back to her right away. The doctor has not done a physical on Jimmy for over a year and he tells the parent that Jimmy needs to come in to be seen. The parent insists!

Reframe. **Adjust your mindset.**	The physician adopts a positive mindset, thinking, "She just has a lot on her mind and a visit would be inconvenient. She's not out to ruin my day."
The Hard Conversations Model	
Step ❶: **Upfront, state your positive intent first.**	"I want to be sure Jimmy is in good health for camp, so he won't have a problem and you can rest easy."
Step ❷: **Tell the truth fast.**	"Someone from our team, whether it's one of my partners, our Nurse practitioner or I, needs to see him in person to check him out. Then, we can be sure he really is in good shape for camp."
Step ❸: **Listen and understand.**	"I realize it might be inconvenient for you to bring Jimmy in, and I'm sorry about the inconvenience. Still, he does need to come in."
Step ❹: **Find common ground.**	"We both want Jimmy to have a great camp experience."
Step ❺: **Identify options and your action plan.**	"I can arrange for our Nurse Practitioner Amanda Berger to see Jimmy at 4 o'clock. Or I personally can see Jimmy tomorrow after school. What will work best for you?"
Step ❻: **Express appreciation.**	"Thanks for understanding and for working with me on this."

This Hard Conversations Model is a blueprint for constructively initiating the hard conversation.

For an excellent model that addresses further complexities of hard conversations, see the comprehensive Courageous Conversations™ Model developed by Judy Dubin and Beth Page of the Cramer Institute.

But What If the Person Resists?

Of course, in practice, hard conversations don't always go so smoothly! People say things like:

- "I can't believe this!"
- "You're off-base."
- "I won't accept that."
- "This is your problem, not mine."
- "You can't be serious!"
- "There are very good reasons for this."
- "You have a point, but…"
- "I won't take NO for an answer."
- "This is ridiculous."
- "No way."

First, listen and see if the person has a point. If you can in good conscience accommodate the person, do so. But if the responsible and appropriate thing to do is to hold your ground, then use the **Caring Broken Record**. This technique enables you to hold your ground without becoming defensive, frustrated or angry. And it saves you time because you avoid getting hooked into endless debates as the other person raises one point after another to push you to change your mind.

 Rule of Thumb 3: Address resistance with the Caring Broken Record.

The Caring Broken Record enables you to hold your ground with caring in the face of resistance ---and not become defensive.

The Caring Broken Record: Three Elements

- Your clear, bottom-line message
- Caring–lots of caring
- And repetition of your message

Your clear, bottom line message is your main point or statement of common ground. State that clearly.

Then comes caring. Mix your bottom line message with lots of caring. For instance, express empathy or acknowledge the person's feelings, as you proceed to hold firm on your main message.

And **repeat yourself**. For as long as the other person resists or persists, keep combining your bottom line message with caring, instead of getting hooked into debating each point the person is making.

For example, in the situation described above, what if the parent wouldn't take NO for an answer and kept insisting that the doctor complete Jimmy's camp form without Jimmy being seen by anyone from the practice? Listen to two contrasting ways the physician can handle this resistance:

Approach 1:

The parent resists. The physician tries to persuade the parent by countering each point the parent makes. The physician gets hooked into debating and becomes defensive.

Parent: "But it's impossible for us to come in! We only have two days left before camp and I must get the form completed!"

Physician: "Well, we can fill out the form only if you bring Jimmy in to be seen."

Parent: "There is no time for him to come in!"

Physician: "I'm willing to accommodate you under this short notice by setting him up to see our Nurse Practitioner."

Parent: "That won't work. He can't come in to see anyone. There is no time."

Physician: "Well, I wish you had planned ahead for this, so there wouldn't be this pressure."

Parent: "Look, my family has been using you for many years and I'm asking this as a favor this one time."

Physician: "I appreciate your family coming here for care, but Jimmy still needs to come in. I don't want to be responsible for clearing him medically without seeing him. What if he then has a problem at camp? I would have committed malpractice."

Parent: "That's not going to happen. He's perfectly healthy and there's no reason why you need to examine him."

Physician: "I hope you're right, but without examining him, we can't be sure."

Parent: "I'm telling you, he is FINE! Can you please just fill out the form?"

Physician: "Not without seeing him. He hasn't been here for over a year, and that's our policy!"

…and on and on…. with both parties becoming very frustrated and their relationship withering.

An alternative approach that works better: *The Caring Broken Record*. This enables the physician to hold his ground without getting frustrated or trying to win a debate with the parent. Here's how the conversation might go if the physician were to use the Caring Broken Record with Jimmy's mother.

Approach 2:

The parent resists and the physician uses the Caring Broken Record.

Parent balks: "But it's impossible for us to come in! We only have two days left before camp and I must get the form completed!"

Physician: "I'm sorry you're under such pressure. Still, Jimmy will need to come in so we can fill out his camp form."

Parent: "Look, my family has been using you for many years and I'm asking this as a favor this one time."

Physician: "I appreciate the opportunity to provide care for your family. Still, to be responsible about Jimmy's health and clear him for camp, one of my partners or I do need to see him."

Parent: "That's not going to happen. He's perfectly healthy and there's no reason why you need to examine him."

Physician: "I realize it's frustrating and inconvenient for you to bring him in especially since you're convinced he's perfectly healthy. Still, I want to be sure, and you will need to bring him in."

More often than not, the parent will come around, not feeling happy about it, but not feeling that the physician was disrespectful or defensive.

Notice that when you handle resistance with the Caring Broken Record, you can shorten the discussion.

Use all three elements of the Caring Broken Record:

* Be clear about your bottom-line message.
* Persist in expressing caring throughout the conversation.
* And convey your bottom-line message with caring over and over until the other person realizes that you are not changing your mind.

The Caring Broken Record helps you reduce the stress of difficult conversations and more often get the results you want. And that's true whether you want to insist on a curfew for your teenager, or handle the myriad tough situations you face with patients and coworkers.

Now, turn the tables.

What if someone initiates a hard conversation with YOU?

Rule of Thumb 4: When you're on the receiving end, open your mind.

- Shake off defensiveness.
- Assume the person is speaking up because they care.
- Open your mind, listen and reflect.

Think to yourself:

- *"Breathe. Listen. I might learn something of value."*
- *"This person cares enough to speak up."*
- *"I can listen without agreeing or disagreeing, and decide later whether to act on what I hear."*

And express your appreciation to the person for caring enough to speak up or share their feedback. For instance:

- *"I'm hearing you and I'll definitely consider what you're saying."*
- *"Thanks for telling me. I know you have our patients' best interest at heart."*

Wrap-Up

Whether you're the initiator or the target, hard conversations are inevitable. When you handle them with courage, skill and respect, everyone wins. The bottom line for hard conversations? *Turn up the warmth--and you'll turn down the heat.*

Highlights for Review: Hard Conversations

Rule of Thumb 1: Beforehand, adjust your mindset to a positive, or at least a neutral one. Shake off frustration or blame and adopt an attitude of respect, openness and inquiry.

Rule of Thumb 2: Follow the Hard Conversations Model

Step ❶: **State your positive intent.**	Explain your purpose, highlighting the benefit to the other person. E.g., *"I want a good relationship with you."*
Step ❷: **Tell the truth fast.**	• Don't beat around the bush. Spill the beans right away. • Be factual and specific. • Explain impact: Consequences and results.
Step ❸: **Listen and understand.**	• Invite reactions and inquire. • Listen intently; acknowledge the person's feelings. • Check your understanding.
Step ❹: **Find common ground.**	• Summarize your shared interest or goal. E.g., *"We both want...."*
Step ❺: **Identify options and your action plan.**	• Identify various ways to proceed and the pros and cons of each. • Agree on your approach – a plan of action for both of you.
Step ❻: **Express appreciation.**	Convey positive regard---thanks, admiration, or appreciation. E.g. *"This wasn't easy, and I appreciate your openness."*

Rule of Thumb 3: If the other person resists, use the **Caring Broken Record**.
- Make your main point with clarity and caring.
- Repeat in the face of continuing resistance.

Rule of Thumb 4: When you're on the receiving end, open your mind.

Selected References

1. Back AL, Communicating bad news. **Western J Med**; Volu. 176;May, 2002: 177-180.

2. Back AL and Arnold RM, Dealing with conflict in caring for the seriously ill: "It was just out of the question". **JAMA**;2005;293(11):1374-81.

3. Back AL et al., Approaching difficult communication tasks in oncology. **CA Cancer. J Clin**;2005;55:164-77.

4. Dubin J and Page B, Courageous Conversations ™; Cramer Institute; www.cramerinstitute.com under "Cramer Institute- Our Programs". Accessed October 24, 2012.

5. Fallowfield L and Jenkins V, Communicating sad, bad and difficult news in medicine. **LANCET**; 2004:Jan 24;363(9405):312-9.

6. Girgis J et al., Breaking bad news: Consensus guidelines for medical practitioners. **J Clin Oncol**;1995;13:2449-2456.

7. Halpern J, Empathy and Patient-Physician Conflicts. **J Gen Intern Med**;2007 May;22(5):696-700.

8. Jain A and Ogden J, General practitioners' experiences of patients' complaints: Qualitative study. **BMJ**. 1999;318:1596-9.

9. Maguire P and Pitceathly C, Managing the difficult consultation. **Clin Med**; 2003;3(6):532-7.

10. McCord RS et al., Responding effectively to patient anger directed at the physician **Fam Med**; 2002;34(5):331-6.

11. Ptacek JT and McIntosh EG, Physician challenges in breaking bad news. **J Behavioral Med**; 2009 ; 32:380-387.

Self-Improvement Tools: Hard Conversations

- **Personal Spot Check**
- **Patient Feedback**
- **Family Feedback**
- **Peer/Colleague Feedback**

Self-Check on a Hard Conversation with a Colleague or Patient	YES ✓
1. I approached the person in a positive, or at least neutral frame of mind.	
2. I started with a positive statement of my hope or purpose for the conversation.	
3. I made my point quickly, instead of beating around the bush.	
4. I listened with an open mind to the other person's point of view.	
5. We agreed on a plan for moving forward.	
6. If the other person became resistant, I remained caring in my manner.	
7. I expressed my appreciation to the other person for hearing me out.	

What did I do particularly well?

What do I want to do differently to improve my approach in the future?

Patient Feedback: On a Hard Conversation

Debrief with the patient after having a hard conversation with them. Perhaps your patient complained to you about something or was frustrated when you held your ground in the face of a request or demand. Or, perhaps you were in a position to deliver bad news. At the end of the conversation, ask them to debrief with you about how you handled the conversation. This will give you the opportunity to address loose ends with this patient and also to learn from the process, so you can handle hard conversations in the future more effectively.

SUGGESTED QUESTIONS

1. *"This was a hard conversation and I appreciate your having it with me. Tell me, at this point, how are you feeling about it?"*

2. *"What else do we need to discuss so you feel better about it?"*

3. *"What did I do or say during this conversation that you felt was helpful?"*

4. *"What did I do or say during this conversation that was not helpful?"*

5. *"Did I check to make sure you felt clear about what we discussed?"*

6. *"What suggestions do you have about how I could have handled our conversation in a better way?"*

Listen well, probe for further information, and end by thanking the person for being open with you about this.

Family Feedback: On a Hard Conversation

Debrief with the patient's family members after they:

- Listened while you held a hard conversation with their loved one
- Participated in a hard conversation involving you and their loved one
- Participated in a hard conversation with you without the patient being present

Ask them to talk with you about how the conversation went for them and how you handled it. This will give you the opportunity to address loose ends, to engage with them more effectively in the future, and also to learn from the process, so you can handle hard conversations with others more effectively.

SUGGESTED QUESTIONS
1. *"This was a hard conversation and I appreciate your being there/engaging with me. Tell me, at this point, how are you feeling about it?"*
2. *"What else do we need to discuss so you feel better about it?"*
3. *"What did I do or say during this conversation that you felt was helpful?"*
4. *"What did I do or say during this conversation that was not helpful?"*
6. *"What suggestions do you have about how I could have handled the conversation in a better way?"*

Listen well, probe for further information, and end by expressing your appreciation for the candid feedback.

 Peer/Colleague Feedback: On a Hard Conversation

Debrief with your colleague after a hard conversation together. Make sure you clear the air and can move forward without resenting each other. Also, learn from this situation so you can handle future hard conversations more effectively.

SUGGESTED QUESTIONS
1. *"My relationship with you is important to me. This was a hard conversation and I appreciate your engaging with me. Tell me, at this point, how are you feeling about it?"*
2. *"What else do we need to discuss, so we can move forward?"*
3. *"What did I do or say during this conversation that you felt was helpful?"*
4. *"What did I do or say during this conversation that was not helpful?"*
6. *"What suggestions do you have about how I could have handled the conversation in a better way?"*

Listen well, probe for further information, and end by encouraging the person to speak up at any time with other thoughts or concerns that will help you work more effectively together.

10. Going Forward

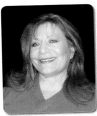

A Letter from Carla Rotering, MD

Dear Colleagues:

Medicine is entering a new era. We as physicians find ourselves perched at the very edge of change - facing unanticipated shifts and transitions that may seem to render the future unpredictable, complex and unknown. We have been expected to participate in new delivery systems, new reimbursement formulas, pay-for-performance systems, complicated regulation, and more–all with the potential to throw us into a reactive mode with the risk of diverting our focus and energies away from our patients.

These changes reflect genuine attempts to shape a new, more effective paradigm for health care – one that embraces excellence and financial prudence – all for the sake of a patient experience that diffuses suffering, connects deeply, and enhances healing on all levels.

It is true that processes, skills and paradigms will support us in facing this transition with professionalism and integrity. What is more true is that it is our human presence – the caring actions of the people of Medicine – that faithfully infuse the patient experience with richness and meaning. We as physicians reside at the heart of the matter. We are the courageous instruments of change, the creative vital force that can transform our hospitals and clinics and all of our places of work with the wisdom to make this new paradigm flourish for patients and for ourselves – every day in every exam room, waiting room, hallway, at every bedside. We are the answers we have been seeking – the people who show the way to a new and better Medicine.

In this Guide, we've condensed for you evidence-based practices that reliably produce the optimal patient and family experience–an experience that is heartwarming, empowering, reassuring and healing. We've also provided growth tools for self-evaluation and for soliciting feedback from others.

These practices and tools can help us respond to the pressures and new rules by elevating our scores on patient experience/satisfaction surveys and maximizing pay-for-performance. More importantly, they provide a way for us to be a strong, positive force in how Medicine is changing. We can use this Guide to achieve personal growth and to re-engage with our noble purpose. We can become activists in the new paradigm of patient and family-centered care and lead the way through our own example.

As I revisited best practices while writing this Guide, I discovered I had a rhythm to my own daily work that fell short, despite a measured pride in my professional excellence and in my fierce advocacy for each and every patient, each and every day. I realized, for instance, that I had never given a minute's thought to how to close an encounter so my patients would feel confident, cared about and special -- with a sense of closure and clarity about next steps. I was used to closing an often deep and intimate encounter with, "Okay, that's it. The nurse will be in to tell you what to do next." And I would dart out to see my next patient. I suddenly became aware that such an abrupt departure might not only leave patients unclear about next steps, but might also leave them feeling diminished and dismissed. I absolutely didn't want that experience for my patients. I certainly didn't want that experience for myself. That awareness opened me to a new level of honesty within myself – an honesty that supported me as I began to look at the places I could improve in my work and an honesty that offered me the courage to change.

I hope you'll join me in using this Guide as a gateway to your own useful insights, as an entry to your own honest inventory that not only illuminates any behaviors that might invite your attention, but also serves as a revolution of optimism that continues to disperse and expand day by day. I hope you'll use the Rules of Thumb, the Self-Assessments, and the Feedback Tools to grow, to refresh, to fine-tune, to excel as you become more powerfully effective in your encounters with patients, families and coworkers. I hope that engaging in this program serves to strengthen the spirit with which you go about your daily work, and offers you a calm certainty that the future of Medicine is safe in our hands and in our hearts.

By opening ourselves to personal improvement and excellence, we emerge as inspirational leaders and exemplars in patient and family-centered care. That is where – and how – we will even more authentically express who we truly are – caring, kind, compassionate people dedicated to enhancing every life we have the privilege to touch. That is the solid ground upon which we walk, now in this present moment and forward toward our hope-filled future.

Kindly,

Carla

Appendix

A: Comprehensive Reference List

The Communication Solution

1. Bartlett G et al., Impact of patient communication problems on the risk of preventable adverse events in acute care settings. **CMAJ**;2008;178(12):1555–1562.

2. Beach MC et al:Relationship-centered care: A constructive reframing. **J Gen Med**;- Jan, 2006:21;Suppl 1:S3-8.

3. Beach MC et al., Is the quality of the patient-provider relationship associated with better adherence and health outcomes for patients with HIV? **J Gen Intern Med**;2006;June:21(6)661-5.

4. Beach MC et al., Do patients treated with dignity report higher satisfaction, adherence, and receipt of preventive care? **Ann Fam Med**;July-Aug;3(4):331-8.

5. Beckman HB et al. The doctor–patient relationships and malpractice: lessons from plaintiff depositions. **Arch Intern Med;**1994;54:1365–70.

6. Bendapudi NM et al., Patients' perspectives on ideal physician behaviors. **Mayo Clin Proc**;2006;81:338–44.

7. Best M and Rosenstein A, Combating physician stress, H and H Daily;4/12/12; Hay Group, **2010 Physician Compensation Survey**.

8. Di Matteo, MR, Enhancing patient adherence to medical recommendations. **JAMA**;1994;271:79-83.

9. Essential Elements of Communication in Medical Encounters: The Kalamazoo Consensus Statement;**Acad. Med**;2001;76:390 – 393.

10. The total package: A skillful, compassionate doctor. **Science Daily**;1/22/09

11. Julliard K et al., What Latina Patients Don't Tell Their Doctors;**Annals of Family Medicine**;Nov/Dec. 2008.

12. Levinson W et al., Developing physician communication skills for patient-centered care. **Health Affairs**;29:7(2010):1310-1318.

13. Levinson W et al., Physician–patient communication: The relationship with malpractice claims among primary care physicians and surgeons. **J Am Med Assoc**;1997;277:553–9.

14. Lewin SA et al., Interventions for providers to promote a patient-centered approach in clinical consultations. **The Cochrane Database of Systematic Reviews**;2001;issue 4.

15. Mauksch LB et al., Relationship, communication and efficiency in the medical encounter: Creating a clinical model from a literature review. **Archives Intern Med.**;2008;168(13):1387-1395.

16. Pacific Business Group on Health, A CQC Guide to Improving the Patient Experience. **California Quality Collaborative;2011**;San Francisco, CA. Available at: http://www.calquality.org/documents/Improving_Pt_Experience_ Spread_Change_Pkg.pdf. Accessed: October 24, 2012.

17. Pandhi N et al., A comfortable relationship: A patient-derived dimension of ongoing care, **Family Medicine**;April 2004.

18. Ptacek JT et al., Quality monitoring of physicians: Linking patients' experiences of care to clinical quality and outcomes. **J Gen Int Med**;2008.

19. Pollak K et al., Physician empathy and listening: Associations with patient satisfaction and autonomy. **JABFM**;2011;24;6:665-672.

20. Rao JK et al., Communication interventions make a difference in conversations between physicians and patients: A systematic review of the evidence. **Med. Care**;2007;45(4);340-9.

21. Roter D, Patient-centered communication. **BMJ**;June 2004.

22. Roter DL and Hall JA, **Doctors Talking with Patients/Patients Talking with Doctors: Improving Communication in Medical Visits**. Praeger:Westport, CT;2006.

23. Roter DL et al., Effectiveness of interventions to improve patient compliance: A meta-analysis. **Med Care**;1998 Aug;36(8):1131-61.

24. Safran DG et al., Switching doctors: Predictors of voluntary disenrollment from a primary care physician's practice. **J Fam Practice**;2000;50(2):130-136.

25. Saha S et al., Patient-centered, cultural competence and healthcare quality. **JAMA**; Nov, 2008.

26. Shanafelt TD et al., The physician-patient relationship and quality of life: Lessons from chronic lymphocytic leukemia. **Leuk Res**;2009;33:263-70.

27. Shanafelt TD et al., Burnout and self-reported patient care in an internal medicine residency program. **Ann Intern Med**;2002;136:358-67.

28. Shortell S, An empirical assessment of high-performing medical groups: Results from a national study. **Medical Care Research and Review**;2005;62(4):407-34.

29. Stagg EV, Incentive plans playing bigger role in physician earnings. **Amednews**; October 4, 2010. Accessed October 24, 2012.

30. Stewart MA, Effective physician–patient communication and health outcomes: a review. **Can Med Assoc J**;1995;152:1423-33.

31. Stewart M et al., The impact of patient-centered care on outcomes. **J Fam Pract**;2000;49:805-7.

32. Sutcliffe KM et al., Communication failures: An insidious contributor to medical mishaps. **Acad Med**;79:186-194.

33. Teal CR and Street RL, Critical elements of culturally competent communication in the medical encounter: A review and model. **Soc Sci Med**;2009 Feb;68(3):533-43.

34. Witherington EM et al., Communication gaps and read- missions to hospital for patients aged 75 years and older: observational study. **Qual Saf Health Care**;2008;17(1):71-75.

35. Zolnerik and DiMatteo, Physician communication and patient adherence to treatment. **Medical Care**;April 2007.

Mindful Practice

1. Davidson RJ and Kabat-Zinn J, Alterations in brain and immune function produced by mindfulness meditation. **Psychosomatic Medicine**;2003;65:564-570.

2. Dunn PM and Arnetz BB, Meeting the imperative to improve physician well-being: Assessment of an innovative program. **J Gen Intern Med**;2007;22:1544-52.

3. Erica MS and Wu A, Clinician mindfulness and patient safety. **JAMA**;2010;304(22):2532-2533.

4. Greeson JM, Mindfulness research update 2008. **Complementary Health Practice Review**;2009;14(1):10-18.

5. Hassed C and de Lisle S, Enhancing the health of medical students: Outcomes of an integrated mindfulness and lifestyle program. **Adv Health Sci Educ Theory Pract**;2009:14(3):387-98.

6. Jensen PM and Trollope-Kumar K, Building physician resilience. **Can Fam Physician**;2008 May;54(5):722–729.

7. Korones DN, Living in the Moment. **JCO**;2010;28(31):4778-4779.

8. Krasner MS et al., Association of an educational program in mindful communication with burnout, empathy, and attitudes among primary care physicians. **JAMA**;2009;302(12):1284-1293.

9. Ludwig DS et al., Mindfulness in medicine. **JAMA**;2008;300(11):1350-1352.

10. Shanafelt T, Enhancing meaning in work: A prescription for preventing physician burnout and promoting patient-centered care. **JAMA**;2009 Sep 23;302(12):1338-40.

11. Shapiro SL and Carlson LE, Mechanisms of mindfulness. **J Clin Psych**;Volume 62, Issue 3;March 2006:373–386.

12. Shapiro S L and Astin J, Mindfulness-based stress reduction for health care professionals: Results from a randomized trial. **International Journal of Stress Management**;Vol 12(2);May 2005:164-176.

13. Swayden KJ et al., Effect of sitting vs. standing on perception of provider time at bedside: A pilot study. **JGIM**;20 (8):677-682;Department of Nursing, University of Kansas Hospital, Kansas City, KS 66160, USA.

14. Wang P and Gao F, Mindful communication to address burnout, empathy, and attitudes. **JAMA**;2010;303(4):330-331.

Mindful Practice and Use of Technology with Patients

1. Frankel RA et al., Effects of exam-room computing on clinician-patient communication: A longitudinal qualitative study. **Patient Educ Couns**;2012 Feb;86(2):166-71.

2. Gold J, Hospitals warn smartphones could distract doctors, March 26, 2012; http://m.npr.org/news/front/149376254?singlePage=true. Accessed October 24, 2012.

3. Margalit RS et al., Electronic medical record use and physician-patient communication: An observational study of Israeli primary care encounters. **Patient Educ Couns**;2006 Apr;61(1):134-41.

4. Nagy V and Kanter M, Implementing the electronic medical record in the exam room: The effect on physician-patient communication and patient satisfaction. **Perm J**;2007 Spring;11(2):21–24.

Collaboration and Teamwork

1. Cleary PD, A hospitalization from hell: A patient's perspective on quality. **Ann Intern Med**;2003;138(1):33–9.

2. Ellingson L, Communication, collaboration and teamwork among health care professionals. **Communication Research Trends**;Centre for the Study of Communication and Culture;V21 (2002);No. 3.

3. Fagin C, Collaboration between nurses and physicians: No longer a choice. **Academic Medicine**;1992:67(5), 295-303.

4. Joint Commission, Behaviors that undermine a culture of safety. **Sentinel Event Alert**;40:July 9, 2008.

5. Larson, E, The impact of physician-nurse interaction on patient care. **Holistic Nursing Practice**;1999:13(2),38-46.

6. Leape L et al., Perspective: A culture of respect, part 1: The nature and causes of disrespectful behavior. **Acad Med**;2012;87:845–852.

7. Leape L et al., Perspective: A culture of respect, Part 2: Creating a culture of respect. **Acad Med**;22 May, 2012.

8. LeTourneau B, Physicians and nurses: Friends or foes? **Journal of Healthcare Management**;2004:49(1),12-14.

9. Lindeke L et al., Nurse-physician workplace collaboration. **OJIN: The Online Journal of Issues in Nursing**;10(1), Manuscript 4.

10. Malone G AND Morath J, Pro-patient partnerships. **Nursing Manage-ment**;2001:32(7);46-47.

11. Milligan R et al., Developing a shared language: Interdisciplinary communication among diverse health care professionals. **Holistic Nursing Practice**;1991;13(2), 47-53.

12. Nairl DM et al., Frequency of nurse–physician collaborative behaviors in an acute care hospital. **J Interprofessional Care**;2011:1–6.

13. Pronovost P et al., Improving communication in the ICU using daily goals. **J Crit Care**;2003;18(2):71-5.

14. Ross A et al., **Interprofessional Relationships and Collaborative Working: Encouraging Reflective Practice. Online J Issues in NSG**;10(10);2005.

15. Sexton J B, et al., Error, stress, and teamwork in medicine and aviation: Cross sec-tional surveys. **Brit Med J**;2000;320(7237):745–9.

16. Stein L et al., Sounding board: The doctor-nurse game revisited. **The New England Journal of Medicine**;1990:322(8):546-549.

17. Sternas K et al., Nursing and medical student teaming for service learning and partnership with the community: An emerging holistic model for interdisciplinary education and practice. **Holistic Nursing Practice**;1999;13(2):66-77.

18. Van Norman G, Interdisciplinary team issues. **Ethics in Medicine**;University of Washington, April 11, 2008.

19. Zwarenstein, M and Reeves S, Working together but apart: Barriers and routes to nurse-physician collaboration. **The Joint Commission**;2002:28(5):242-247.

20. Zwarenstein M & Reeves S, Knowledge translation and interprofessional collaboration: Where the rubber of evidence-based care hits the road of teamwork. **Journal of Continuing Education in the Health Professions**;2006:26, 46–54.

21. Zwarenstein M et al., Interprofessional collaboration: Effects of practice-based interventions on professional practice and healthcare outcomes. **Cochrane Database of Systematic Reviews** 2009;Issue 3;No CD000072.

Effective Openings and Closings

1. Bakic NM, Successful doctor-patient communication and rapport-building as the key skills of medical practice. **Medicine and Biology**;2008;(15)2:74–79.

2. Frankel R and Stein T, Getting the most out of the clinical encounter: The Four Habits model. **Permanente J**;Fall 1999;3:3.

3. Halpern J, Gathering the patient's story and clinical empathy. **Permanente J**;Winter 2012:16:1.

4. Langewitz W et al., Spontaneous talking time at start of consultation in outpatient clinic: cohort study. **BMJ**;2002 Sep 28;325(7366):682-3.

5. Ness DE et al., Language and connectedness in the medical and psychiatric interview. **Patient Educ & Couns**, 2007;68(2):139-144.

6. Robinson JD, Closing medical encounters: Two physician practices and their implications for the expression of patients' unstated concerns. **Social Science & Medicine**; 53 (2001):639–656.

7. Roter DL, Communication patterns in the primary care interview. 1997;**JAMA**;277(4):350-6.

8. Scannell D, Narrative medicine: A case of baffling fatigue with a spectral twist; **Permanente J**; Winter 2012:Vol. 16, No. 1.

9. Stein TS and Kwan J, Thriving in a busy practice: Physician-patient communication training. **Eff Clin Pract**; 1999;2(2):63-70.

Engaging Patients and Their Families as Partners

1. Barry M, Shared decision-making: Informing and involving patients to do the right thing in health care. **J Amb Care Man**;(2012):35, 2, 90-98.

2. Bieber C. et al., Training physicians in shared decision-making-who can be reached and what is achieved. **Patient Education and Counseling**;2008:77(1),48-54.

3. Beach MC et al., Do patients treated with dignity report higher satisfaction, adherence and receipt of preventive care? **Annals of Family Medicine**;3(4); Jul/Aug 2005:331-338.

4. Berwick DM, What patient-centered should mean: Confessions of an extremist. **Health Aff**;(Millwood) 2009;28:w555-w565.

5. Blanchard J and Lurie N, R-E-S-P-E-C-T: Patient reports of disrespect in the health care setting and its impact on care. **J Fam Pract**.;2004;53:721-730.

6. Coleman MT and Newton KS, Supporting self-management in patients with chronic illness. **Am Fam Physician**;2005;(72)8:1503-1510.

7. Coulter A, **Engaging Patients in Health Care**. 2011;NY: McGraw-Hill Education.

8. Coulter A et al., Effectiveness of strategies for informing, educating and involving patients. **BMJ**;2007:335(7609),24-27.

9. Fowler FJ et al., Informing and involving patients to improve the quality of medical decisions. **Health Affairs**;2011;390, 699-706.

10. Frankel R et al., Crossing the patient-centered divide: Transforming health care quality through enhanced faculty development. **Academic Medicine**;2011; 86 (4):445.

11. Frosch D. et al., Authoritarian physicians and patients' fear of being labeled 'difficult' among key obstacles to shared decision making. **Health Affairs**; No. 5 (2012):1030–1032.

12. Gordon T, Edwards WS, **Making the Patient Your Partner: Communication Skills for Doctors and Other Caregivers**. Auburn House: Westport CT;1997.

13. Greenfield S et al., Expanding patient involvement in care. Effects on patient outcomes. **Ann Intern Med**;1985 Apr;102(4):520-8.

13. Hanson JL, Have we missed the obvious? **Archives of Int Med**;2008;168:1368-1370.

14. Holman H, Lorig K. Patients as partners in managing chronic disease. **BMJ**;2000;320:526-527.

15. Institute for Healthcare Improvement, **Delivering Great Care: Engaging Patients and Families as Partners**. 2006. Available at www.IHI.org. Accessed October 24, 2012.

16. Joffe S et al, What do patients value in their hospital care? An empirical perspective on autonomy centred bioethics. **J Med Ethics**;2003;29;103-108.

17. Lysaught MR, How respect for persons became respect for autonomy. **J Med Philos**;2004;29:665-680.

18. Michaud MD et al., Ten strategies to build partnerships with patients. **Wisconsin Med J**;2007;106, 8:444-446.

19. Moumjid N et al., Shared decision making in the medical encounter: Are we all talking about the same thing? **Medical Decision Making**;2007;27:539-546.

20. Murray E et al., Clinical decision-making: Patients' preferences and experiences. **Patient Education and Counseling**;2007;65:189-196.

21. Parchman ML et al., Participatory decision making, patient activation, medication adherence, and intermediate clinical outcomes in type 2 diabetes. **Ann Fam Med**;2010;8:410–7.

22. Peikes D et al., Patient-Centered Medical Home Decision Maker Brief. Rockville, MD: **Agency for Healthcare Research and Quality**, February 2011, PP11-51.

23. Rask KJ et al., Patient activation is associated with healthy behaviors and ease in managing diabetes in an indigent population. **Diabetes Educ**;2009 Jul-Aug;35(4):622-30.

24. Rollnick S et al., Motivational interviewing. **BMJ**;2002;340:1242-1245.

25. Scholle, SH et al., Engaging Patients and Families in the Medical Home. **Agency for Healthcare Research and Quality**;Rockville, MD;June 2010:Document No. PR10-24. 73 Pages.

26. Street Jr RL, et al., Patient participation in medical consultations: Why some patients are more involved than others. **Med Care**;2005;43:960–9.

27. Patients as partners: How to involve patients and families in their own care. **Joint Commission Resources**;2006.

28. Wilson SR et al., Better outcomes of asthma treatment (BOAT) study group. Shared treatment decision making improves adherence and outcomes in poorly controlled asthma. **Am J Respir Crit Care Med**;2010;181:566–77.

Communicating with Empathy

1. Back A et al., **Mastering Communication with Seriously Ill Patients: Balancing Honesty with Empathy and Hope**. New York: Cambridge Univ Pr;2009.

2. Bonvicini KA et al, Impact of communication training on physician expression of empathy in patient encounters. **Patient Education and Counseling**;2009: 75(1), 3-10.

3. Branch WT Jr et al., A good clinician and a caring person: Longitudinal faculty development and the enhancement of the human dimensions of care. **Acad Med**;2009;84: 117–25.

4. Churchill LR and Schenck D, Healing skills for medical practice. **Ann Intern Med**;2008;149:720-4.

5. Coulehan JL et al., Let me see if I have this right: Words that help build empathy. **Ann Intern Med**;August 7, 2001:135:221-227.

6. Decety J, Empathy in clinical practice. In **Empathy: From Bench to Bedside** (Social Neuroscience). Cambridge, MA:MIT Press;2011:229-244.

7. Easter DW and Beach W, Competent patient care is dependent upon attending to empathic opportunities presented during interview sessions. **Curr Surg**;2004;61:313-8.

8. Fadiman A, **The Spirit Catches You and You Fall Down: A Hmong Child, Her American Doctors, and the Collision of Two Cultures**. NY: Farrar, Straus and Giroux;1997.

9. Fogarty LA et al., Can 40 seconds of compassion reduce patient anxiety? **J Clin Oncol**;17:371-379.

10. Frenkel DN and Liebman CB, Words that heal. **Ann Int Med**;140(6):482-483.

11. Halpern J, Empathy and patient-physician conflicts. **J Gen Intern Med**;2007; 22:696-700.

12. Hojat M et al., Physicians' empathy and clinical outcomes for diabetic patients. **Acad Med**;2011;86:359-64.

13. Kim SS et al., The effects of physician empathy on patient satisfaction and compliance. **Eval Health Prof**;2004;27:237-51.

14. Levinson W et al., A study of patient clues and physician responses in primary care and surgical settings. **JAMA**;2000;284:1021-7.

15. Makoul G, Essential elements of communication in medical encounters: the Kalamazoo consensus statement. **Acad Med**;2001;76:390-3.

16. Mercer SW and Reynolds WJ, Empathy and quality of care. **Br J Gen Psychiatry**;2002;52(9-12).

17. Morse DS et al., Missed opportunities for interval empathy in lung cancer communication. **Arch Intern Med**;2008;168:1853-8.

18. Moyer CA et al., What factors create a humanistic doctor? A nationwide survey of fourth-year medical students. **Acad Med**;2010;85:1800-7.

19. Rainer S et al., Physician–patient communication in the primary care office: a systematic review. **J Am Board Fam Pract**;2002;15:25–38.

20. Rakel DP et al., Practitioner empathy and the duration of the common cold. **Fam Med**;2009;41:494-501.

21. Schattner A, Who cares for empathy? **QJM**;2012;105(3):287-290.

22. Schattner A, The silent dimension. Expressing humanism in each medical encounter. **Arch Intern Med;2009**;169:1095-9.

23. Stepien KA and Baernstein A, Educating for empathy. **J Gen Intern Med**;2006; 21:524-30.

24. Suchman AL et al, A model of empathic communication in the medical interview. **JAMA**;1997;Feb 26;277(8):678-82.

Effective Explanations

1. Casarett D et al., Can metaphors and analogies improve communication with seriously ill patients? **J Palliative Care**;13(3).

2. Boyle CM. Differences between patients' and doctors' interpretation of some common medical terms. **BMJ**;1970;1:286–289.

3. Britten N et al., Misunderstandings in prescribing decisions in general practice: qualitative study. **BMJ**;2000;320:484–8.

4. Castro CM et al., Babel babble: physicians' use of unclarified medical jargon with patients. **Am J Health Behav**;2007;31(Suppl 1):S85–S95.

5. Davis TC et al., The gap between patient reading comprehension and the readability of patient education materials. **J Fam Pract**;1990;31:533–538.

6. Flacker J et al., Hospital discharge information and older patients: do they get what they need? **J Hosp Med**;2007;2(5):291–296.

7. Gibbs R et al., Patient understanding of commonly used medical vocabulary. **J Fam Pract**;1987;25:176–178.

8. Hewson MG, Patient education through teaching for conceptual change. **J Gen Intern Med**;1993;8:393–8.

9. Kemp EC et al., Patients prefer the method of "Tell Back- Collaborative Inquiry" to assess understanding of medical information. **J Am Board Fam Med**; 2008;21(1):24-30.

10. Kripalani, S et al., Health literacy and the quality of physician-patient communication during hospitalization. **J Hospital Medicine**;Vol 5 (5);2010

11. Kripalani S et al., Promoting effective transitions of care at hospital discharge: a review of key issues for hospitalists. **J Hosp Med**;2007;2(5):314–323.

12. Coleman EA and Berenson RA, Lost in transition: Challenges and opportunities for improving the quality of transitional care. **Ann Intern Med**;2004;141(7):533–536.

13. Kripalani S, Weiss BD, Teaching about health literacy and clear communication. **J Gen Intern Med**;2006;21:888–890.

14. Kripalani S et al., Deficits in communication and information transfer between hospital- based and primary care physicians: implications for patient safety and continuity of care. **JAMA**;2007;297(8):831–841.

15. Logan PD et al., Patient understanding of emergency department discharge instructions. **South Med J**;1996;89:770-4.

16. Institute of Medicine, **Health Literacy: A Prescription to End Confusion**. Washington, DC: National Academies Press;2004.

17. Makaryus A and Friedman E,, Patients' understanding of their treatment plans and diagnosis at discharge. **Mayo Clin Proc**;2005;80(8):991–994.

18. Makoul G, Essential elements of communication in medical encounters: the Kalamazoo consensus statement. **Acad Med**;2001;76:390–3.

19. Mayeaux EJ et al., Improving education for patients with low literacy skills. **Am Fam Physician**;1996;53:205–211.

20. **Medical Oncology Communication Skills Training Learning Modules**; 2002; Available at: http://depts.washington.edu/oncotalk/learn/modules/Modules_01.pdf. Accessed: October 24, 2012.

21. Periyakoil V, Using metaphors in medicine. **J Palliative Med**;11(6), 2008.

22. Pfizer Clear Health Communication Initiative, www.pfizerhealthliteracy.com.

23. Sudore RL et al., Unraveling the relationship between literacy, language proficiency, and patient-physician communication. **Patient Educ Couns**;2009;75(3):398–402.

24. Weiss BD, **Health Literacy: A Manual for Clinicians**. Chicago, IL: American Medical Association;2003.

Hard Conversations

1. Back AL, Arnold RM, Dealing with conflict in caring for the seriously ill: "It was just out of the question". **JAMA**;2005;293(11):1374–81.

2. Back AL et al., Approaching difficult communication tasks in oncology. **CA Cancer. J Clin**;2005;55:164– 77.

3. Fallowfield L and Jenkins V, Communicating sad, bad and difficult news in medicine. **LANCET**;2004;Jan 24;363(9405):312-9.

4. Girgis J et al., Breaking bad news: Consensus guidelines for medical practitioners. **J Clin Oncol**;1995;13:2449-2456.

5. Groves J, Taking care of the hateful patient. N Engl J Med;1978;298;(16):883–7.

6. Halpern, J, Empathy and Patient-Physician Conflicts. **J Gen Intern Med**;2007 May;22(5):696–700.

7. Jain A and Ogden J, General practitioners' experiences of patients' complaints: qualitative study. **BMJ**;1999;318:1596-9.

8. Maguire P and Pitceathly C, Managing the difficult consultation. **Clin Med**; 2003;3(6):532–7.

9. Makadon HJ, Gerson S, Ryback R. Managing the care of the difficult patient in the emergency unit. **JAMA**;1984;252:2585–8.

10. Makoul G et al, Using an online forum to encourage reflection about difficult conversations in medicine. **Patient Education and Counseling**;2010;79(1):83-86.

11. McCord RS et al, Responding effectively to patient anger directed at the physician. **Fam Med**;2002;34(5):331–6.

12. Platt FW and Gordon GH, **The Field Guide to the Difficult Patient Interview**. Lippincott Williams & Wilkins;Philadelphia, 1999.

13. Ptacek JT and McIntosh EG, Physician challenges in breaking bad news. **J Behavioral Med**;2009;32:380-387.

14. Quill T & Townsend P, Bad news: Delivery, dialogue and dilemmas. **Archives Internal Medicine**;1991:151:463-468.

15. Stone D et al., **Difficult Conversations: How to Discuss What Matters Most**. New York, NY: Penguin Books;1999.

Looking Back on Today

SELF-REFLECTION	YES ✓
1. Did I take a deep breath and focus before approaching my patients?	
2. Did I greet my patients warmly and establish positive rapport immediately?	
3. When I was visiting with a patient, did I sit, lean in and adopt an open, receptive posture?	
4. When the patient was speaking to me, did I pay undivided attention, instead of shuffling papers, typing, taking notes, or looking at the computer?	
5. If there were family members present, did I treat them with respect and regard from the start?	
6. Did I express empathy to my patients?	
7. Did I encourage patients to share their feelings?	
8. Did I acknowledge the patient's feelings in an empathetic way?	
9. Did I validate or confirm the legitimacy of the patients' feelings?	
10. Did I show empathy in my nonverbal behavior, by nodding and looking concerned?	
11. If family members were present, did I show empathy for their feelings?	
12. Did I ask the patient how much they want to know and honor their preference?	
13. Did I find out from the patient what they already knew, so I could build on this and address misinformation?	
14. Did I avoid using acronyms and jargon, so patients could easily understand me?	
15. Did I encourage the patient to speak freely about their concerns before I intervened?	
16. Did I invite the patient's ideas and viewpoints before making suggestions?	

SELF-REFLECTION	YES ✓
17. Did I encourage questions as I proceeded with an explanation?	
18. Did I find out what people understood, instead of taking for granted that they understood me?	
19. Did I make a concerted effort to engage the patient in decisions?	
20. When family members were present, did I invite their questions and address their concerns?	
21. Did I check the patient's (and family member's) understanding and comfort with next steps before ending the visit?	
22. When I had bad news to share with a patient, did I plan my approach so I was more likely to handle it well?	
23. Did I make the last six seconds of our interaction a positive memory?	
24. If I had an issue with a colleague's actions, did I address it directly with that person?	
25. Did I acknowledge and appreciate coworkers who were involved in the patient's care?	
26. Did I open my mind to diverse perspectives from others on the care team?	
27. If I had an issue with a coworker, did I raise the issue with this person directly?	
28. If I had an issue with a coworker, did I raise the issue in a caring way?	
29. If I had a hard conversation with a colleague, did I listen with an open mind to the other person's point of view?	
30. If a colleague had an issue with me, did I listen and consider their point of view without being defensive?	
31. Did I communicate well with coworkers about the patient's care, so we would be on the same page and not confuse the patient?	
32. Did I act as a positive role model for collaboration and teamwork?	

Feedback from Patients

In our recent visit:	YES ✓
1. Did I make you feel welcome?	
2. Did I pay good attention to you and your family when we were talking?	
3. Did I make you feel important?	
4. Did I communicate in a respectful way with my coworkers in front of you?	
5. Did I ask you what you hoped to learn from the visit?	
6. Did we address the concerns you most wanted to discuss?	
7. Did I explain things clearly, not using unfamiliar terms?	
8. Did I make a point of encouraging you to ask questions?	
9. Did I check to make sure you felt clear about what we discussed?	
10. Did I involve you in the discussion as much as you wanted?	
11. Before ending, did I check your understanding and comfort with next steps?	
12. If any of our conversation was emotionally hard, did I handle this in a caring way?	
13. Did I make the last six seconds of our interaction a positive memory for you?	
14. Do you feel you could call me if you have a concern later?	

Feedback from the Patient's Family

In our recent visit:	YES ✓
1. Did I make you feel welcome?	
2. Did I pay good attention to you and the patient when we were talking?	
3. Did I listen well?	
4. Do you think I made the patient feel important?	
5. Did I make you feel important?	
6. Did I communicate in a respectful way with my coworkers?	
7. Did I ask you what you hoped to learn from the visit?	
8. Did we address the concerns you most wanted to discuss?	
9. Did I explain things clearly, not using unfamiliar terms?	
10. Did I make a point of encouraging questions?	
11. Did I check to make sure you and the patient felt clear about what we discussed?	
12. Did I involve you in the discussion as much as you wanted?	
13. Before ending, did I check the patient's and/or your understanding and comfort with next steps?	
14. If any of our conversation was emotionally hard, did I handle this in a caring way?	
15. Did I make the last six seconds of our interaction a positive memory for you?	
16. Do you feel you could call me if you have a concern about the patient later?	

Feedback from a Coworker Who Observed
My Behavior with a Patient (and Family)

In the recent visit:	YES ✓
1. Did I greet the patient warmly and by name?	
2. If family members were present, did I make a point of greeting them warmly and introducing myself?	
3. Did I give the patient my undivided attention when we were talking?	
4. Did I avoid letting the computer or other tech device hurt my communication with the patient?	
5. Do you think I acted in a way that made the patient feel important?	
6. If family members were present, did I give them undivided attention when they were talking?	
7. Did I connect with the patient by showing knowledge of them as a person and knowledge of their medical history?	
8. Did I ask the patient to identify all of their concerns before setting an agenda?	
9. If family members were present, did I ask them what they hoped to learn from the visit?	
10. Did we work together to set the agenda for the visit?	
11. Did I appear to address the concerns that mattered most to the patient?	
12. Did I show empathy for the patient's feelings?	
13. Did I find out what the patient already knew, so I could build on this and address misinformation?	
14. Did I avoid using acronyms and jargon, so the patient could easily understand me?	
15. Did I make a point of encouraging the patient to ask questions?	
16. Did I engage the patient in decisions about their care?	
17. Did I check for understanding, instead of taking for granted that the patient understood me?	
18. Before ending, did I check understanding and comfort with next steps?	
19. Did I make the last six seconds a positive memory for the patient?	
20. With the patient, did you think I behaved in a collaborative way?	

Feedback from My Coworkers about My Interactions with Them

About my interactions with coworkers:	YES ✓
1. Do I greet coworkers warmly as if I'm glad to see them?	
2. Do I appear to welcome diverse views and ideas?	
3. Do I communicate with you in a respectful way?	
4. When I hand off a patient or a patient's information to you, do I do so in a way that eases your way with the patient?	
5. Do I make myself available when you and I need to discuss a patient's condition or plan?	
6. Do you think I do my part in making sure you and I are on the same page regarding the patient's care?	
7. Do you think I am respectful in interactions with others on the staff?	
8. If I have a concern with you, do I raise it directly to you in a caring way?	
9. If you have ever given me negative feedback, have I listened without being defensive?	
10. Do you see me as a positive role model for collaboration and teamwork?	

Feedback from a Shadow Coach

If your organization has a Coaching Program for physicians, inquire and request a Shadow Coach. A "Shadow Coach" is typically a non-physician trained to observe a physician from the perspective of a patient, although some physicians simply ask a coworker, a volunteer or even a family member or friend to serve as their Shadow Coach. The Coach joins the physician in a patient visit and observes quietly. Ahead of time, the Coach reviews a Best Practices Checklist to become familiar with what to observe. Then, the person observes the patient-physician interaction. Afterward, the Coach completes the Best Practices Checklist and shares the feedback with the physician. Most physicians who use Shadow Coaches are struck by how helpful the feedback is, and as a result of the feedback, most initiate improvements in their communication methods that result in improved patient experience scores as well.

Best Practices Checklist for Shadow Coach

Best Practices Checklist for Shadow Coach	YES ✓
1. Greeted the patient warmly.	
2. Called the patient by name.	
3. Sat and leaned toward the patient while the patient was talking.	
4. Showed prior knowledge of the patient as a person.	
5. Showed knowledge of the patient's medical history.	
6. If family members were present, introduced self to them as well.	
7. Asked the patient to share all topics he or she wanted to discuss.	
8. Listened to all topics before delving into any one of them.	
9. Negotiated the agenda with the patient, agreeing on what was most important to discuss in this visit.	
10. Listened to patient talk about their concerns without interrupting.	
11. Acknowledged the patient's feelings in an accepting manner.	
12. Followed up on the patient's feelings.	
13. Validated the patient's feelings.	
14. Asked the patient to share what they already knew about each topic, so the physician could build on this.	
15. Clarified how patient could get help later with a concern or question.	
16. Explained things in a way that was easy to understand.	
17. Used the Teach-Back technique to check patient's understanding.	
18. Worked together with the patient to arrive at a plan.	
19. Involved the patient in decisions.	

Best Practices Checklist for Shadow Coach	YES ✓
20. Made a genuine effort to encourage questions.	
21. Inquired about the patient's values and customs and their impact on options being discussed.	
22. Stayed connected to the patient despite use of a computer or other tech device.	
23. Invited family members to ask questions.	
24. Summarized key points and decisions.	
25. Before ending, checked comfort with next steps.	
26. Treated the patient with respect.	
27. Handled difficult issues in a direct and caring way.	
28. Made the last six seconds a positive memory for the patient.	
29. Patient appeared satisfied at the end of the visit.	

Best-Selling Books by Wendy Leebov, Ed.D.

http://www.quality-patient-experience.com/wendy-leebov-books.html

 Physician Entrepreneurs: The Quality Patient Experience -- Improve outcomes, boost quality scores, and increase revenue *(Book and CD-2008)* Built around the key areas in the CAHPS survey, this book and tool-packed CD offers quick and easy techniques that physicians and practice staff can use to enhance the patient experience–without sacrificing productivity.

 Wendy Leebov's Essentials for Great Patient Experiences: No Nonsense Solutions with Gratifying Results *(2008)* Specific tools that enhance the patient experience and address the difficulties staff have in delivering the exemplary care they would like to provide. High-impact strategies for moving your service excellence and patient satisfaction to a new level, resulting in higher scores on HCAHPS and CG-CAHPS.

 Wendy Leebov's Essentials for Great Personal Leadership: No Nonsense Solutions with Gratifying Results *(2008)* Valuable problem-solving and leadership development for health care executives, mid-level administrators, department heads, clinical leaders, and anyone who brings a passion to their work. Each chapter captures the essence of emotionally intelligent leadership and focuses on effective solutions.

 Service Quality Improvement: The Customer Satisfaction Strategy for Health Care *(Leebov and Scott)* A goldmine of approaches for your service excellence initiative, helping you build a service-oriented culture and focusing all employees on service excellence and continuous service improvement.

 The Indispensable Health Care Manager: Success Strategies for a Changing Environment *(Leebov and Scott - 2003 Health Care Book of the Year)* Identifies ten role shifts needed by managers who want to add significant value to their organizations and enhance their employability. Self-assessments, case situations and concrete tools that build key leadership competencies.

Also by Wendy Leebov–practical guides that help frontline employees provide the exceptional patient and family experience

- Assertiveness Skills for Professionals in Health Care
- Customer Service for Professionals in Health Care
- Telephone Skills for Professionals in Health Care
- Resolving Complaints for Professionals in Health Care
- Working Together for Professionals in Health Care

Enrich Your Tools and Confidently Guide Your Team to the Next Level
http://www.quality-patient-experience.com/wendy-leebov-books.html

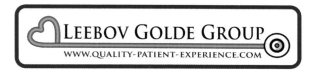

Programs and Services for Physicians, by Physicians

Leebov Golde Group physicians partner with systems, hospitals, health plans and medical practices to provide a remarkable and healing patient experience, while also boosting HCAHPS/CG-CAHPS scores, pay-for-performance and physician satisfaction. How? By helping physicians strengthen and intentionally employ evidence-based best practices for communicating with patients, families and their colleagues on the healthcare team.

Options Tailored to Your Needs

1. The Language of Caring for Physicians: Communication Essentials for Patient-Centered Care

Groundbreaking physician engagement strategy and web-based CME program that:

- Strengthens the important spoken and unspoken conversations that reside between physician, patient and family
- Helps physicians make patient- and family-centered care a reality
- Improves communication and collaboration among all members of the care team
- Improves HCAHPS and CG-CAHPS scores, patient safety and clinical outcomes
- Helps hospitals and physicians optimize earnings under Value-Based Purchasing and pay-for-performance
- Promotes physician satisfaction
- Accomplishes this in a manner that respects physicians' significant time constraints

Strategy options include: Leadership Kickoff, Training of Peer Coaches, Kickstart Session for Physicians, and the Eight-Module, web-based CME program, **The Language of Caring for Physicians**.

2. Strategy for Enhancing Hospitalist Performance

Strengthens the hospitalist team's skills in building relationships and improving communication with patients, families, other physicians and members of the healthcare team. Choose skill-building presentations or implement a customized strategy to achieve breakthroughs in hospitalist performance.

3. Presentations (On-Site and/or via Webinar)

- Skill content tailored to your needs
- Individual sessions or a series
- Popular topics:
  - › HCAHPS, CG-CAHPS and How to Score High
  - › Medicine as Noble Work
  - › From Captain of the Ship to Team Leader

4. Using Coaching to Improve Physician Performance

- Training for physician leaders and peer coaches
- Strategies for instituting peer coaching program

For More Information, Contact:

Jill Golde, Senior VP : 314-571-9607; jgolde@quality-patient-experience.com
Dorothy Sisneros, Senior VP: 602-615-1192; dsisneros@quality-patient-experience.com